THE CARDBOARD HOUSE

LARRY TOWELL

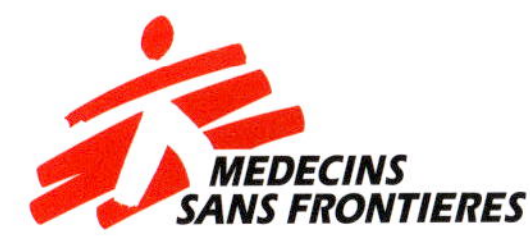

MSF PERU

END OF A MISSION

ACTION ON AIDS

TROLLEY

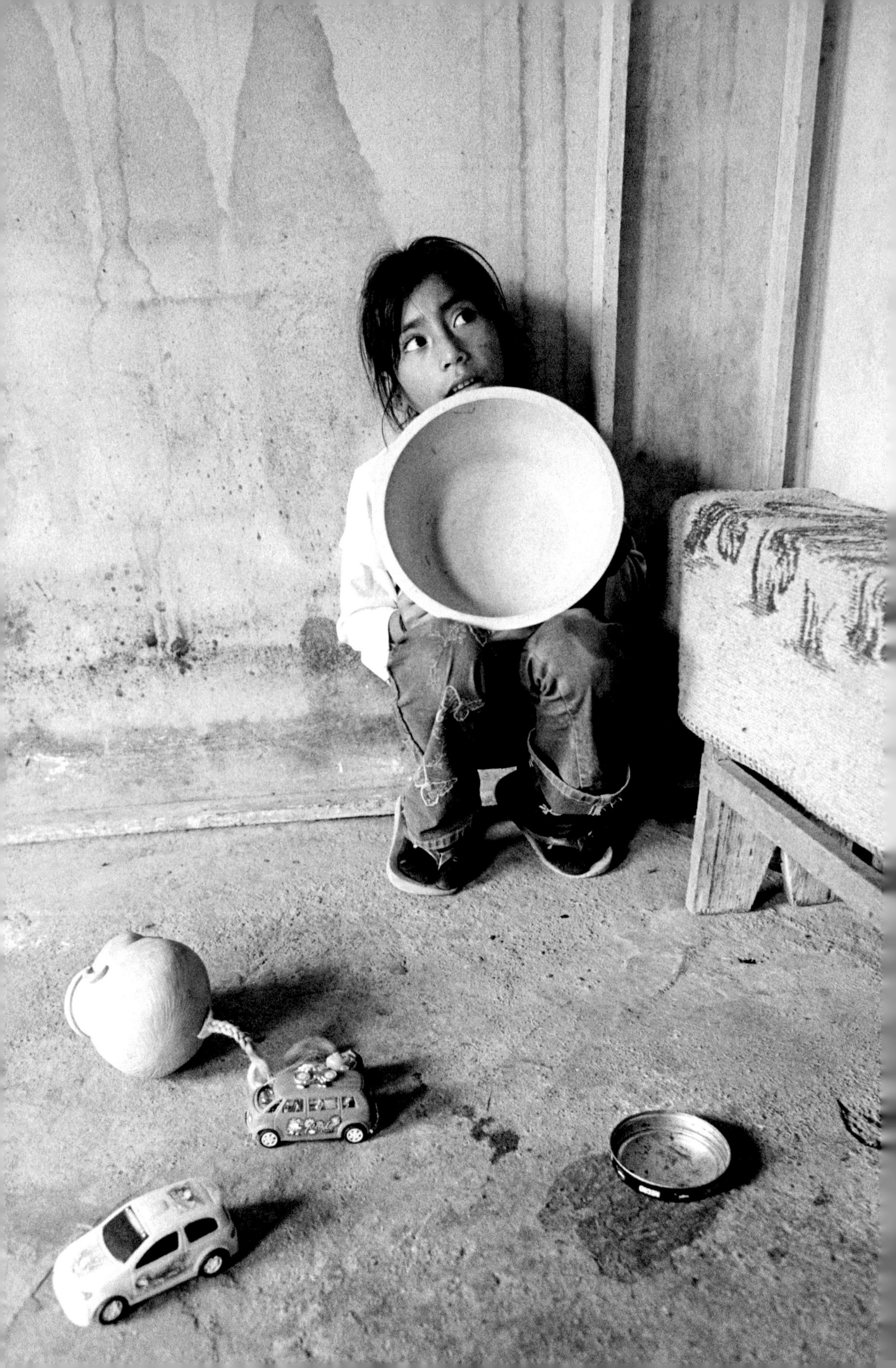

7 PREFACE
PIERO GANDINI

12 WOMEN HIV+ AT HOME
BETTY
GLORIA
ZOILA

34 STREETS
THALIA
MARTINA

50 BROTHEL
ROSA
PATRICIA

68 CHORRILLOS (FEMALE PRISON)
CARMELA
LIZETH

94 LURIGANCHO (MALE PRISON)
IVAN
LUIS ALBERTO
MIGUEL
WONDER WOMAN

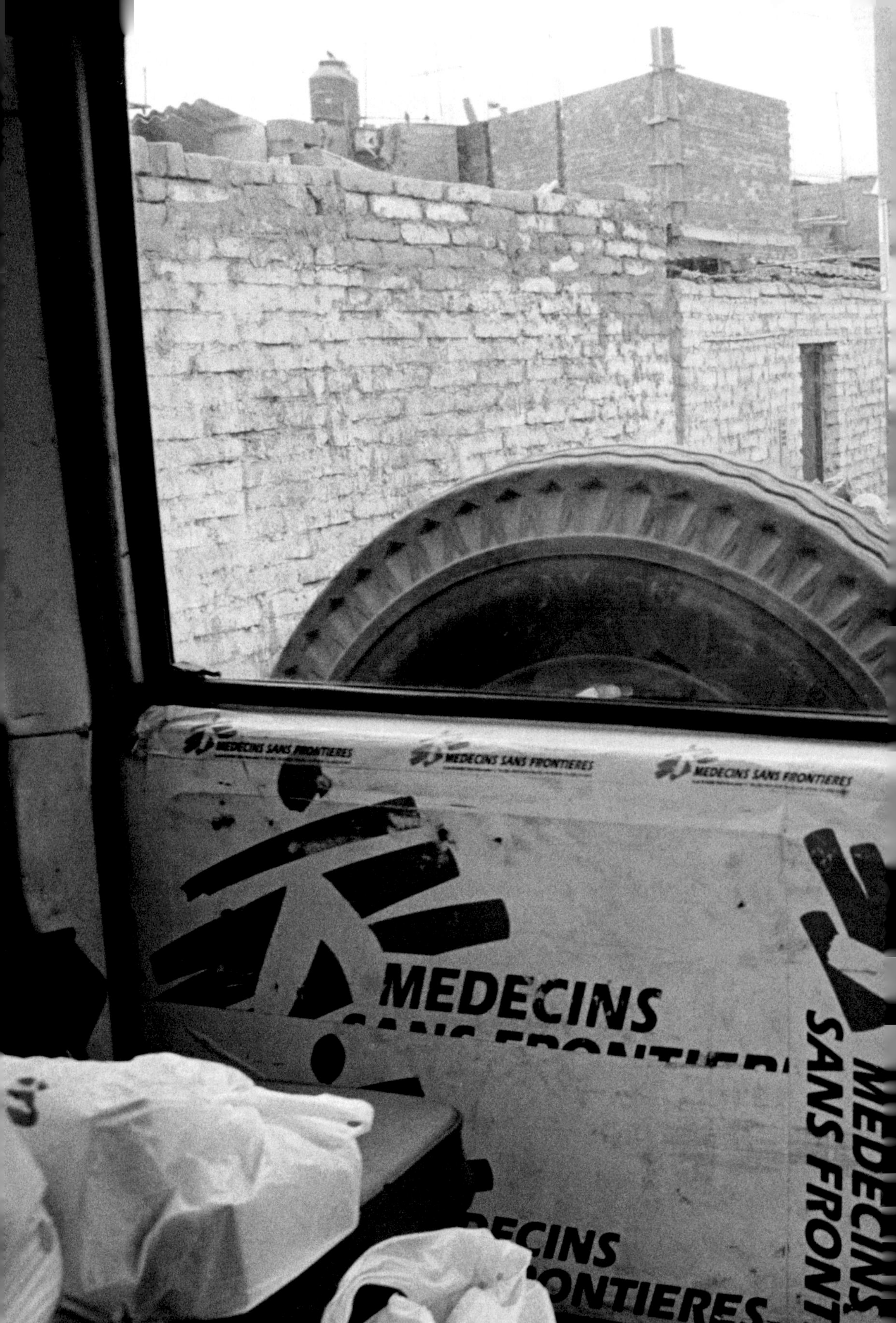
MEDECINS SANS FRONTIERES
MEDECINS SANS FRONTIERES
MEDECINS SANS FRONTIERES
MEDECINS
SANS FRONTIERES
MEDECINS
FRONTIERES
MEDECINS
SANS FRONT

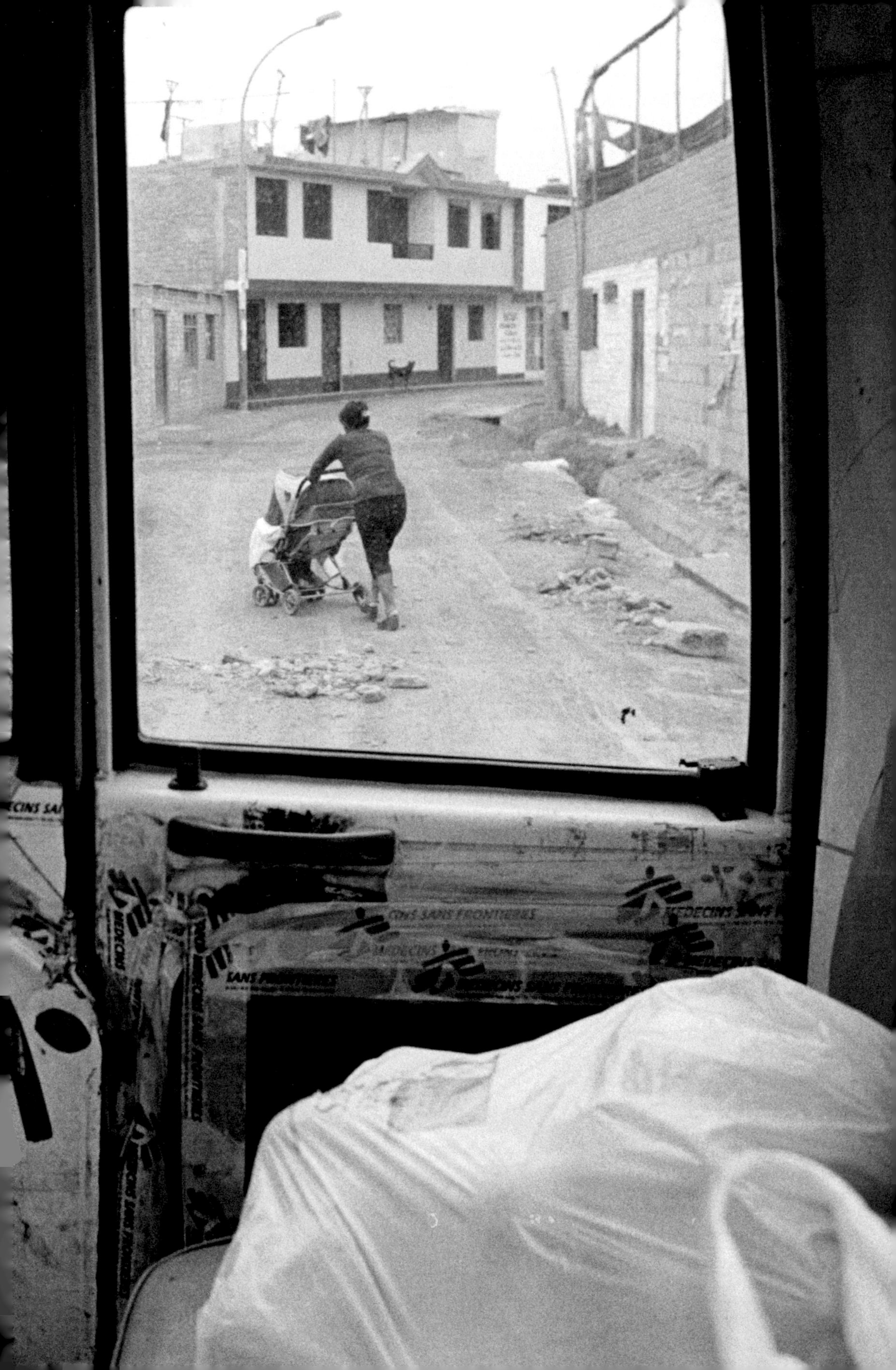

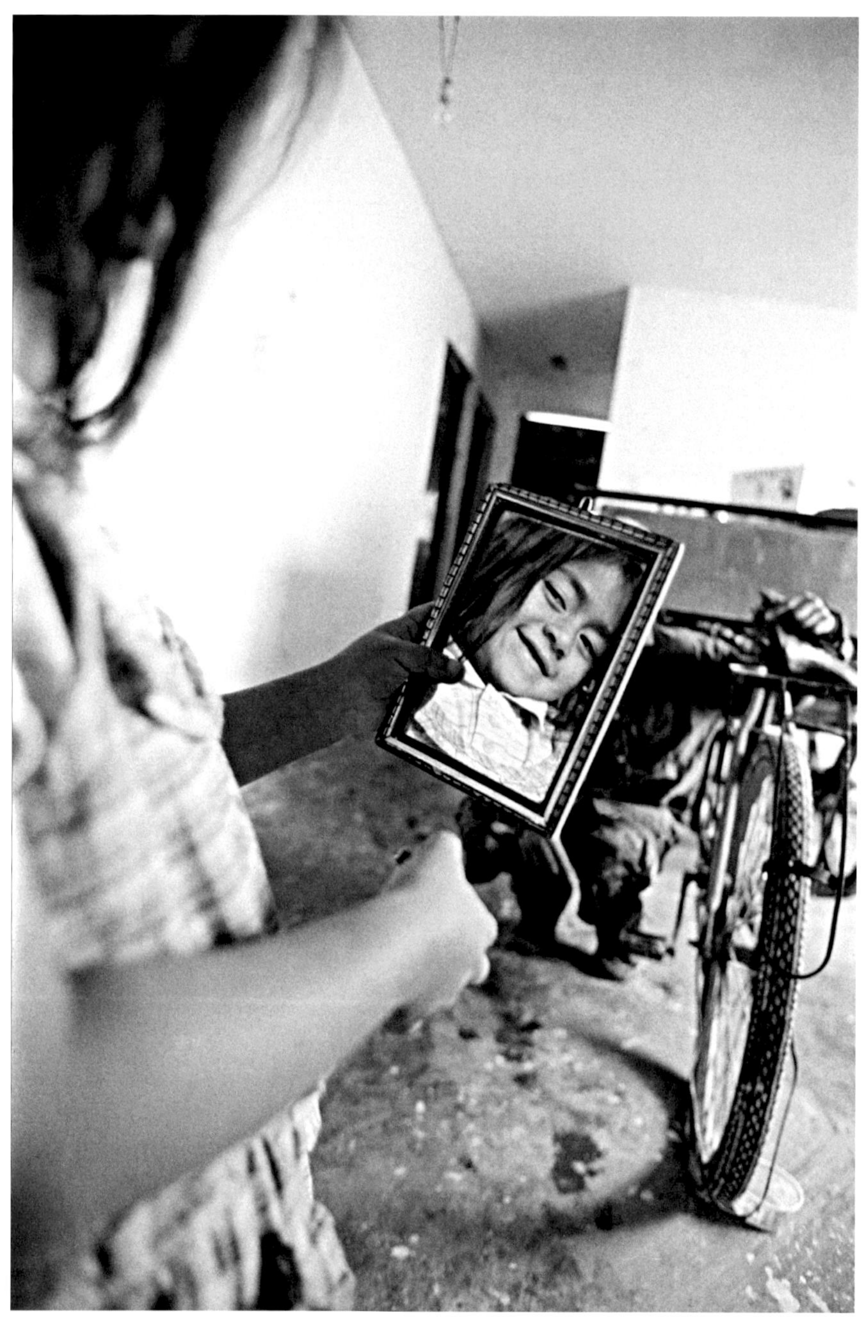

Preface

Piero Gandini
Head of Mission (2005-2007)
MSF Peru

"For those who were forgotten even before they die"
Graffiti in Lurigancho Prison

This is a book about human lives, shunned by the society to which they belong. At the same time it is a simple view, the normal life of normal people, seen through the lens of Larry Towell during his visits to Médecins Sans Frontières (MSF) projects in Lima, Peru. His images emcompass the project for decentralized HIV/AIDS care at a district level in the slum of Villa El Salvador, and the control of Sexual Transmitted Infections (STI) and HIV/AIDS within prisons, including the vast male prison at Lurigancho, and two other prisons in the Lima region.

Peru is considered a low prevalence country in terms of HIV/AIDS (less than 1% are infected), but in specific groups such as commercial and transvestite sex workers, and people deprived of liberty in the prisons, the prevalence is several times higher. These groups have been considered the target population since the mid 1990's for the projects that MSF have implemented in Peru.

Through this remarkable book MSF would like to bring to light some daily aspects of ordinary people that have been rejected and excluded from society, who faced daily difficulties to survive with dignity, and who now feel a sense of empowerment in their lives.

The first chapter shows us women living with HIV/AIDS and involved with the MSF project CATITSS in Villa El Salvador, (a Health and HIV/AIDS Treatment Center of the San José Mother and Children Hospital, built by MSF). The slum of Villa el Salvador is the poorest area of Lima, and probably the whole of Peru. Inhabited by more than half a million people, mainly migrants from other regions in the country, a high percentage of the population are below the poverty line with terrible living conditions, lack of clean water, as well as high crime and unemployment rates. Women here are also subject to high incidences of domestic violence.

These women, along with other women that are HIV positive in Peru, show an example of strength and determination to move their lives forward. The majority of them have been infected by their own husbands or partners, some are already widows and have to take care of their children alone. They are women ready to bring back their quality of life despite being HIV positive, women that every day must fight poverty, prejudice and discrimination. Theirs are stories that teach us the value of love and bravery.

Other images communicate the lives of women who have been able to raise their families, and give education to their sons and grandsons, through working in one of the oldest and most frequented brothels in the Lima-Callao area. Real mothers and grandmothers, every night they face solitude and uncertainty.

Towell also captures the periculous existence of transvestites working on the cold, dark and dangerous streets of Lima, their lives at risk simply to earn a few dollars to survive. Their faces and bodies hide discrimination, persecution and often mistreatment.

Theirs are again real stories full of human suffering and poverty, but also of strength and courage in the face of a hypocritical and uncaring society.

Finally we see the inmates of the female Chorrillos and male Lurigancho prisons. Women and men without freedom, they are denied adequate healthcare, human rights and opportunities. Living in deprivation, they still possess their own diverse realities, dynamics and problems. Chorrillos is divided into two sectors: maximum security, where there are around 250 inmates (mostly former combatants of the rebel group Shining Path), and common, where there are approximately 700 women and 35 children.

Lurigancho prison is the biggest prison in Peru and probably one of the most crowded and dangerous prisons in Latin America. The majority of the men inside Lurigancho prison are still without a proper judiciary process: only 14% of the almost 9,000 inmates have been sentenced, the rest are still awaiting their trials. The situation inside Chorrillos's common sector is different to that in the male prison of Lurigancho. Living conditions are better, there are less people therefore it is less crowded, but they are similarly restricted in terms of healthcare and slow judiciary processes.

Lurigancho prison exists as a sort of society in itself, and encompasses several groups even further outcast and neglected within it: the poor and homeless living in the dump area of the prison, transvestite sex-workers, drug-users and those who are sick, predominantly with Tuberculosis and HIV.

Crude realities, yet nevertheless these photographs and stories describe a sense of empowerment and dignity that has been brought into the lives of these previously forgotten and discriminated people.

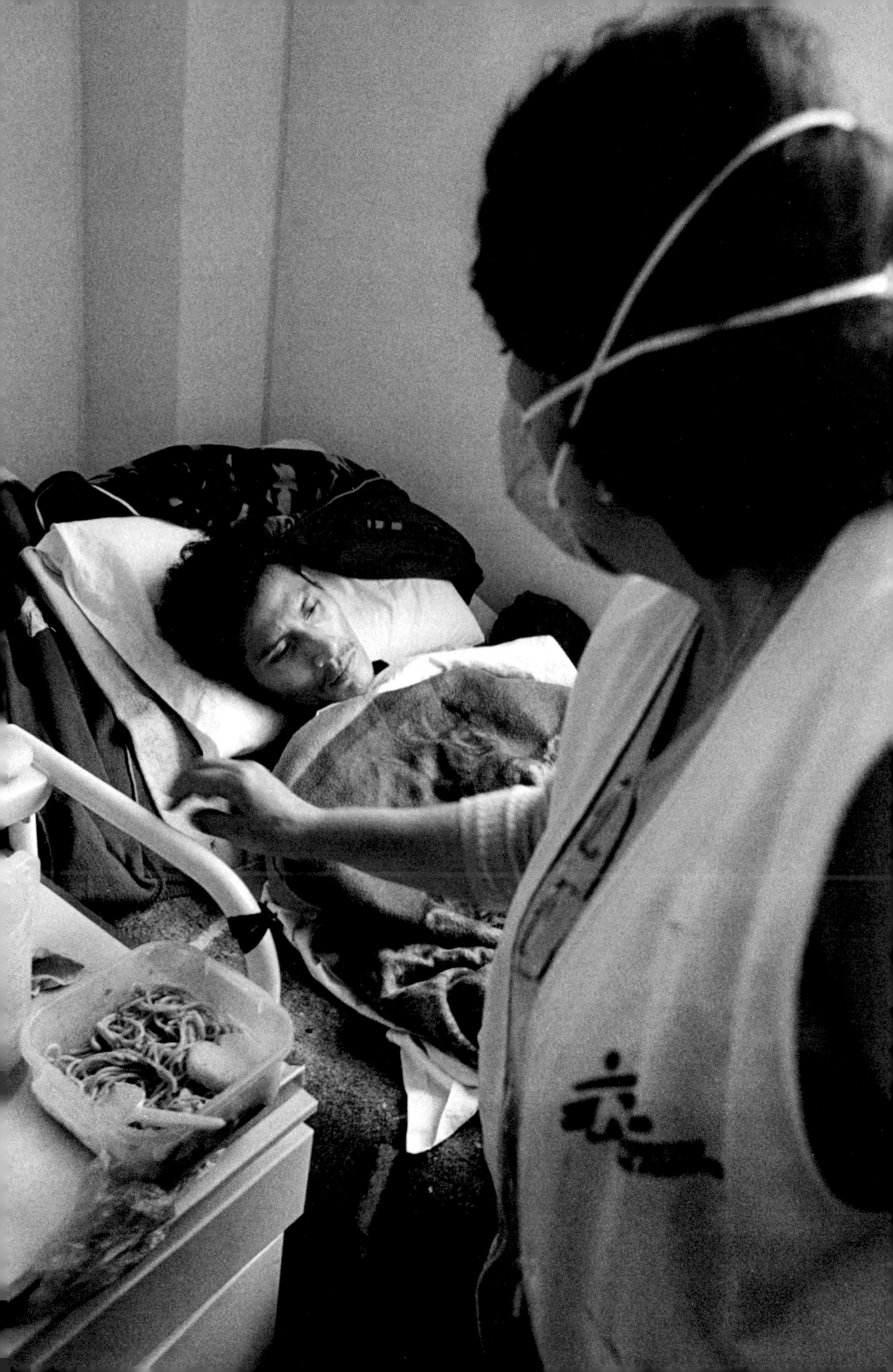

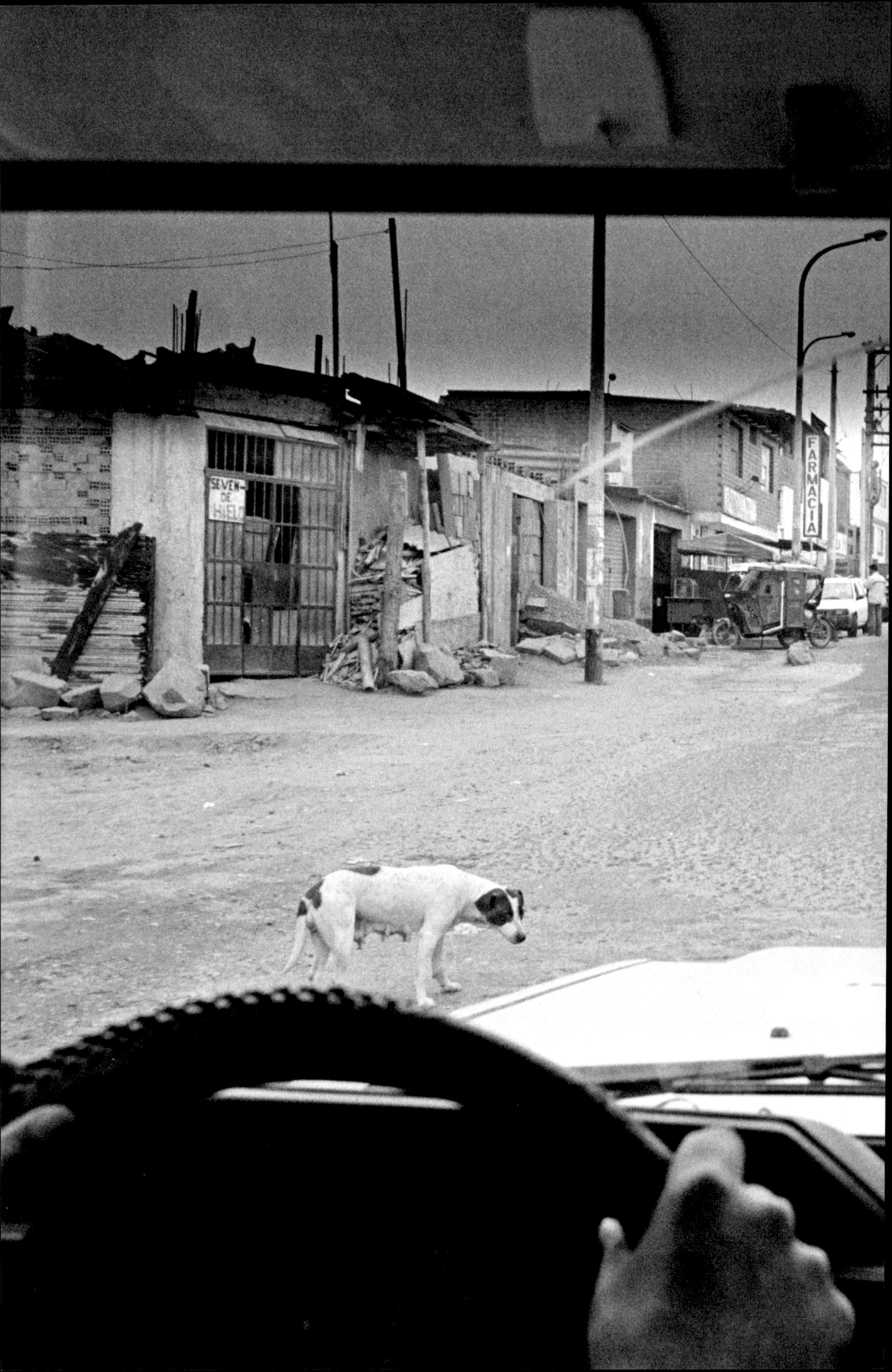
SE VEN-
DE
HIELO
FARMACIA

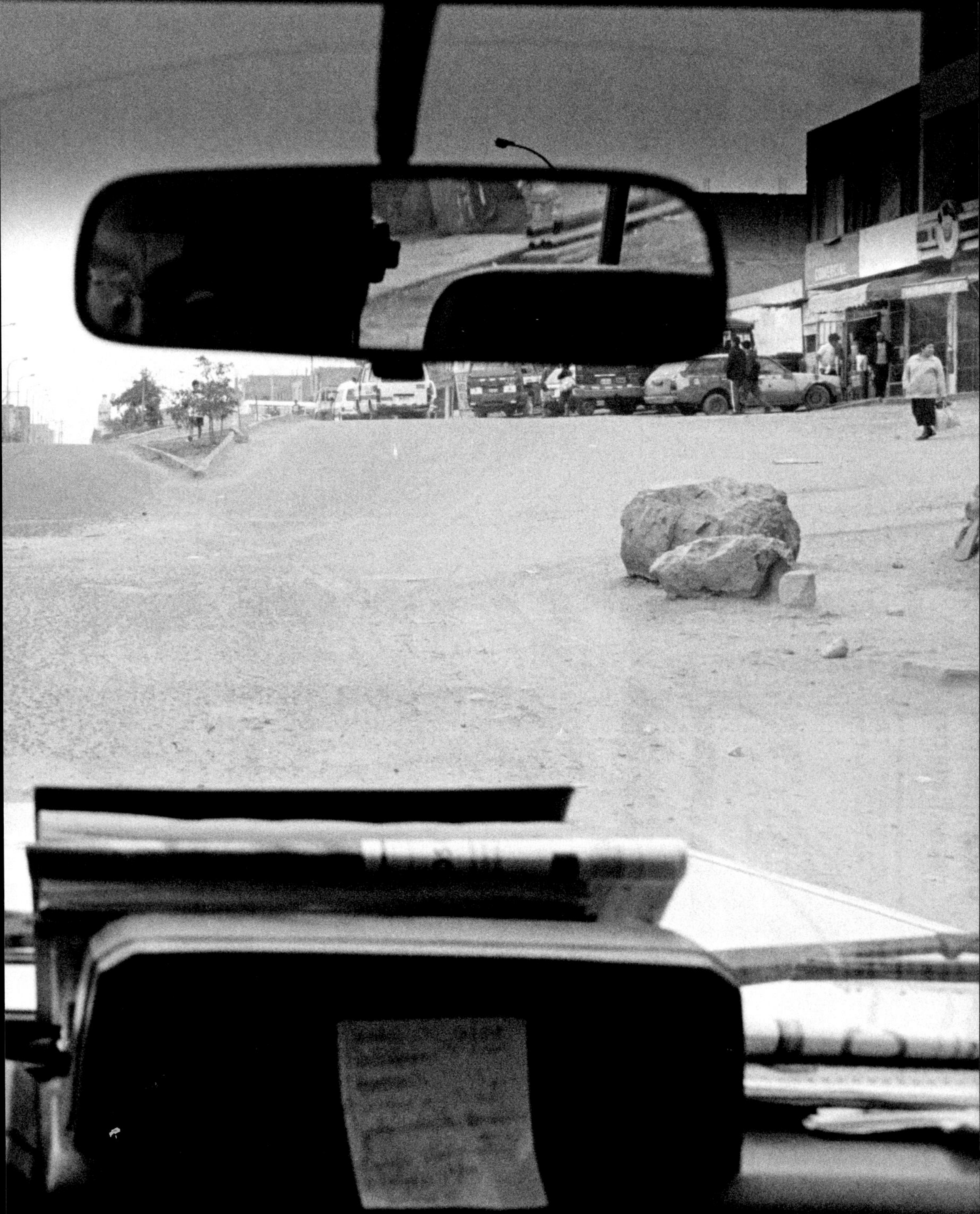

Betty

**HOUSEWIFE AND EMPLOYEE AT THE SAN JOSÉ CATITSS • 26 YEARS OLD
2 DAUGHTERS (5 AND 2), SINGLE MOTHER • LIVES IN VILLA EL SALVADOR
WITH HER MOTHER AND SIBLINGS**

In 2003, I found out I had HIV. I was pregnant with my second daughter and my partner had left me. I don't know how to explain how I felt. I was stunned, I didn't cry or anything. Then I began to think about my daughter, about the baby I was carrying, the worst thoughts came to my mind, that maybe she would be born with deformities or that I would die during labor. But the worst part was that I kept on crying, not because of the diagnosis, but because he had left me! Until one day I said, "Enough. I don't have much time and I shouldn't waste it on a man that only treats me badly."

He was someone who harmed me greatly; he hit me, yelled at me, insulted me in the street. Of course after he would talk to me in a nice way saying, "I love you," and I would fall at his feet, I would melt like butter. Now I think he didn't appreciate me, I was some kind of masochist. Whenever we fought, in the end I always wasted my time going out to look for him. Everything I did was in order to please him or my family… it was just because I needed to have a livelihood, right? To have enough money for food, diapers, two or three treats, and that's all. Then, after I got HIV, how was I going to stay with someone who could leave me at any time or that could get me pregnant again?

My mom, dad, brothers and sisters all know I have HIV, but I don't want to tell my aunts and uncles or neighbors; in the end, this doesn't make me any different or make people love me more or less because I am still the same person. Besides, I don't tell them because of my mother, she tells me, "What are your aunts going to think, that you prostitute yourself?" When I was sick, my mother made up the story that I had cancer, leukemia. I respect her decision, all this must be very hard for her.

I also do it because of my daughters. Here in Villa El Salvador there is a lot of discrimination and fear regarding HIV. If I said, "You know teacher, I have HIV", the first thing they would do is to kick my daughter out of school, they would think she was infected. There was a psychologist at this school and I told her to talk to my daughter a lot. At that time, I thought I wasn't going to last long and I wanted her to talk to my daughter about my brother-in-law and my sister, and tell her that he was her father, because they were going to take care of her. I think she guessed what I had, but said nothing.

Every day, when I see my daughters asleep in their beds, I look at them and say to myself, "How am I going to tell them? How long will I be here? How old will they will be when I get sick?" I don't think it can happen... but I could start feeling ill. I don't want them to suffer, to see me sick. My oldest daughter suspects something. She is 5. She thinks I am sick because she sees me take the pills. She reminds me, "Mommy, your pills, you have to take them or else you'll have a headache." How does she know? I don't know... If my head or back hurts, she lies down beside me and rubs my head, my back. She gets a little scared. She is quite mature, she talks to her little sister and says, "Keep quiet, mom is not feeling well, her head hurts. Let's tidy up." And they begin to fix the house and their things.

I have thought about writing to my daughters, telling them all about my experience, like a diary. Using my own words, in my own hand, telling them what I think, what I would have liked to tell them then, explain to them that I love them, that they mean everything to me, that I am trying hard and that if I am sticking to the treatment it is for them; I would tell them not to become disappointed in me just because I've changed. It would be great to read the diary to them myself when they are older.

As I said before, as a result of the diagnosis and my daughters, I began to think about myself. If before everything boiled down to him, now it was me. I started looking for ways of improving my economic situation. I sold puddings in front of my house, then hair bands, purses and bracelets, which I knitted with my mom. I saved money to buy more materials. "I am planning" I thought, and I liked that. Then I got a cleaning job at the San José CATITSS, where I am currently working. I feel safer, and more willing to better myself. I didn't used to think about the future before, but now I do.

In the future, I see myself with a company, my own house and a car. My new partner has experience in the printing business and we are saving our money. He is a good and cheerful person, he doesn't yell at me and he adores my daughters. We make plans together, "Betty, how much have we saved?" How much will we spend?" With what we have saved we are going to buy a printing machine to print invoices, receipts or cards. He can teach me how to use it, so I can work while he works at the other printing house. I could find customers. And little by little, we could save to buy another machine and save up to buy a piece of land or a house. Having my own company or a house would make me very happy.

We are participating in a GAM (self support group), and together with the other people we are thinking about "getting our acts together" because even with MSF here, there are problems with the Ministry of Health because sometimes they are very fickle. They offer one thing and then they don't fulfill it; for example, there is a constant lack of staff, there is only one assistant nurse and the doctor is always in meetings and people have to wait a long time or return the next day. That is why we are strengthening ourselves, to keep watch when there is not enough staff or treatment and to complain about this shortage if necessary.

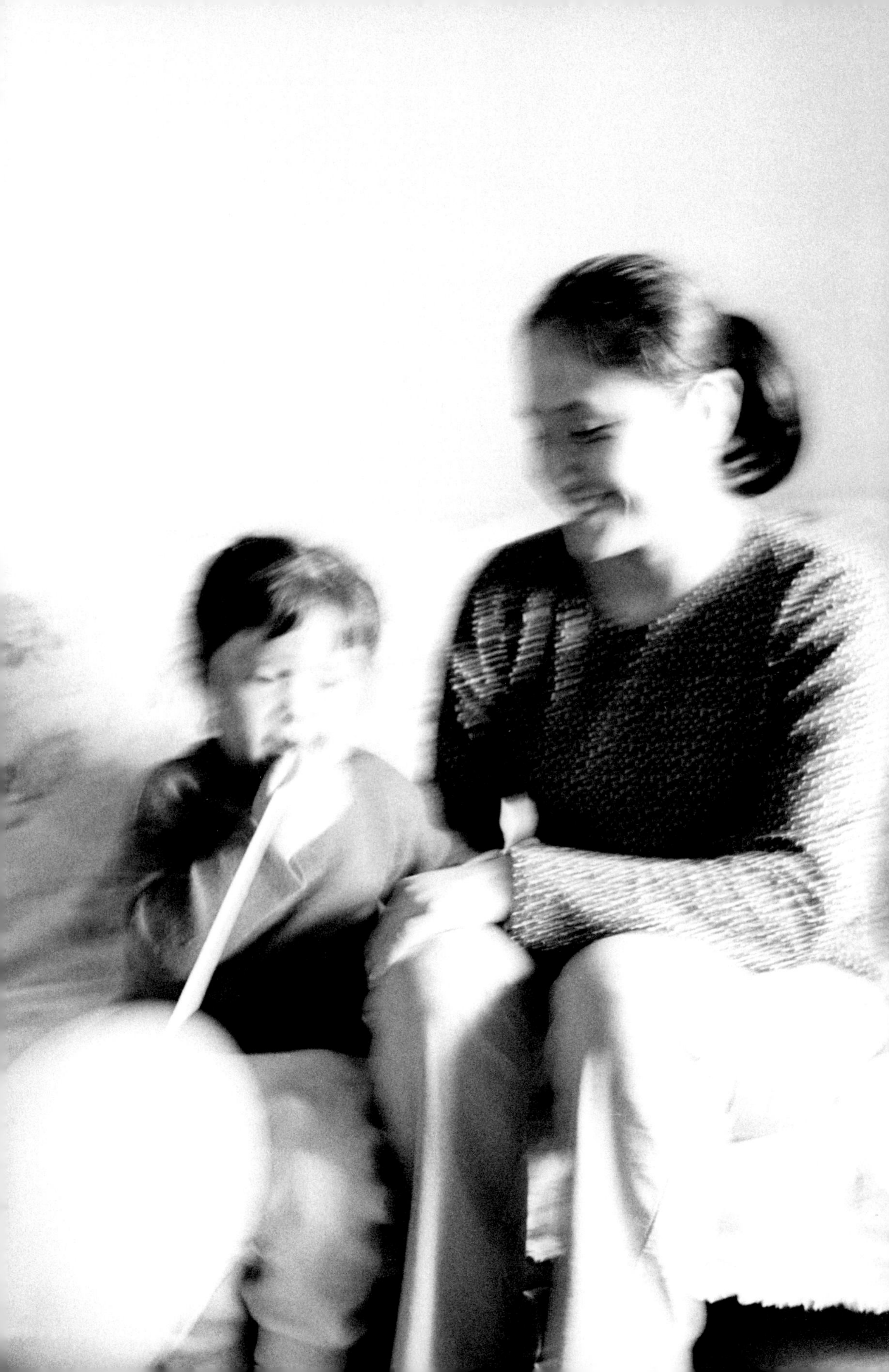

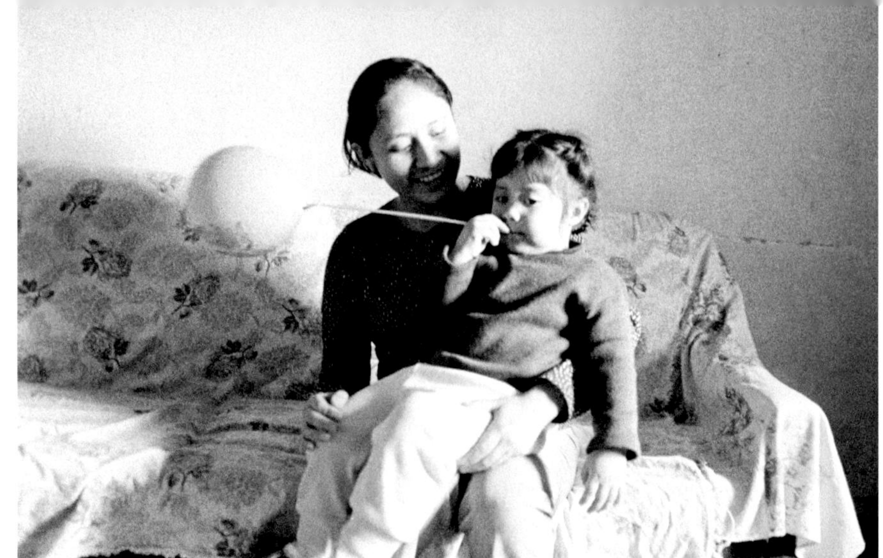

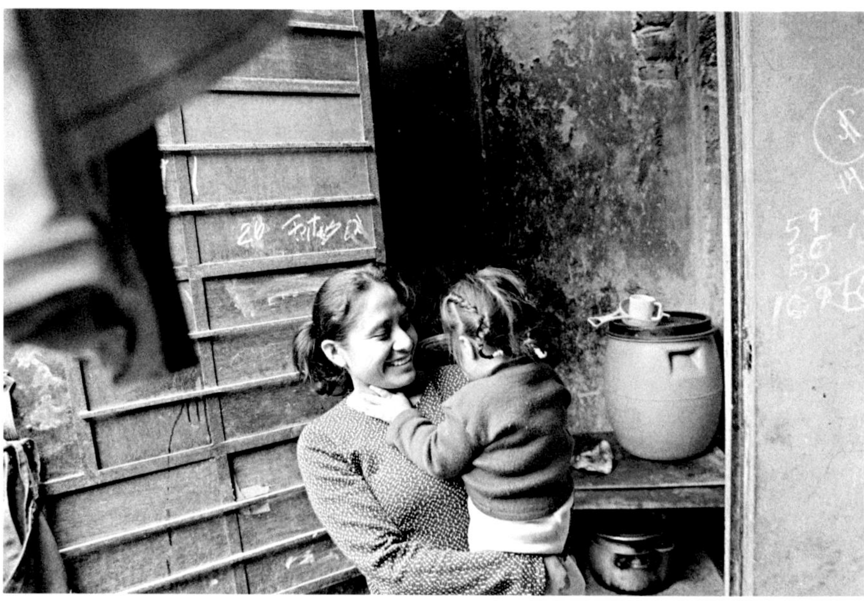

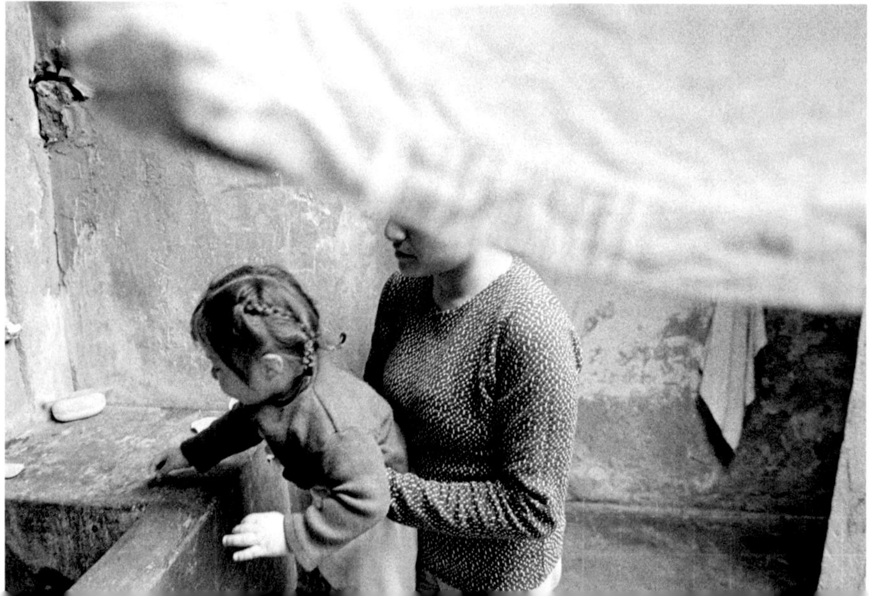

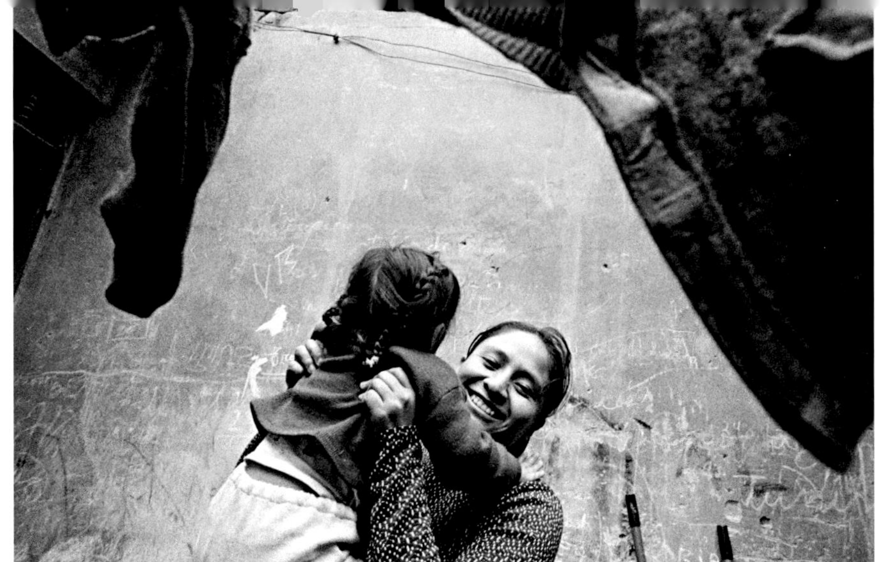

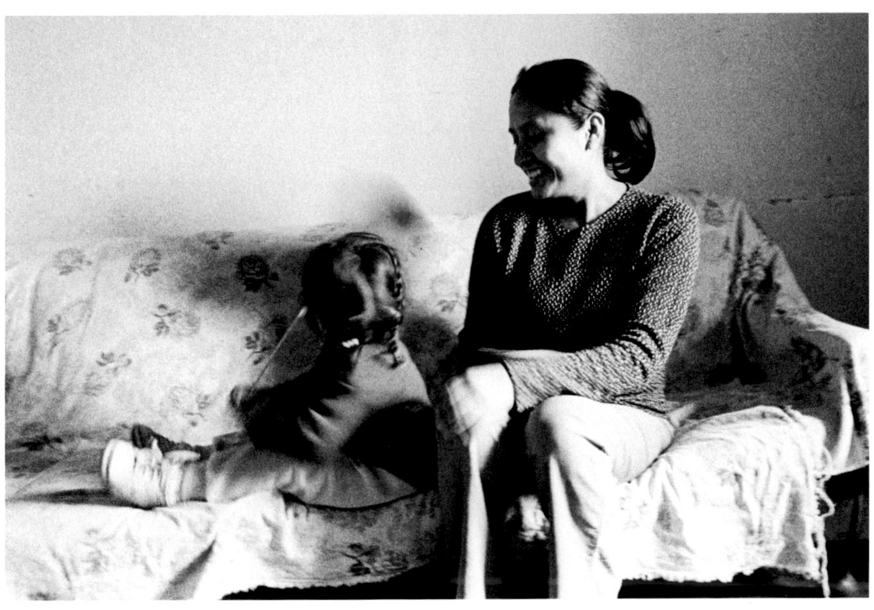

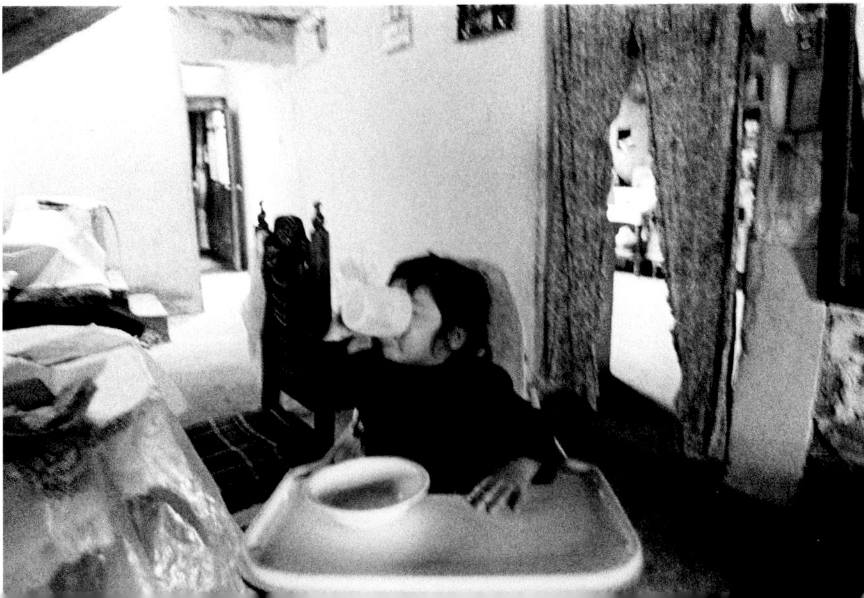

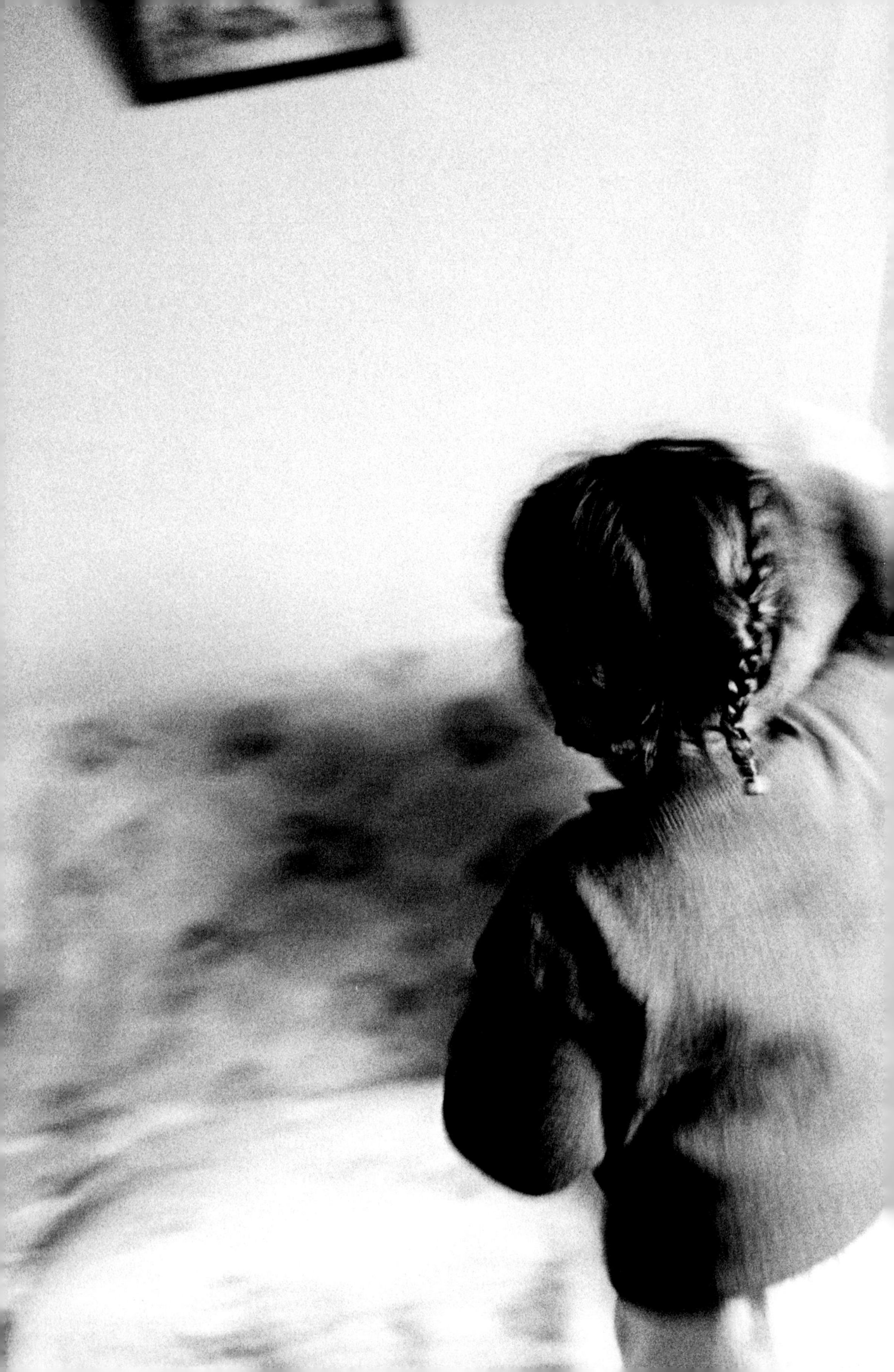

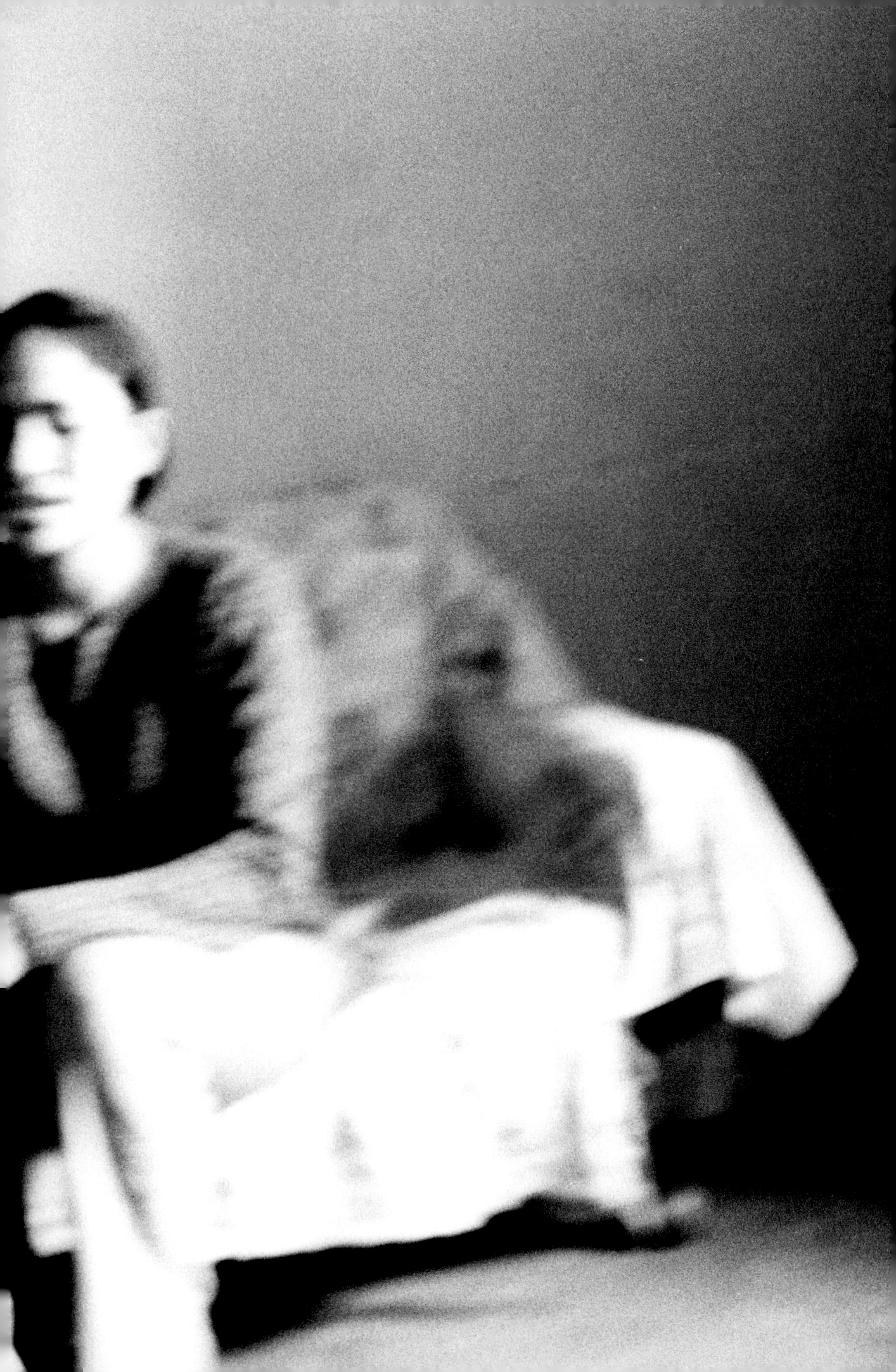

Gloria

HOUSEWIFE • 36 YEARS OLD • 1 DAUGHTER • LIVES IN VILLA EL SALVADOR
USER OF CATITSS

My name is Gloria and I live in Villa El Salvador, one of the poorest districts in Lima. When I was born my family gave me two names: Jenny and Gloria. I've always used Jenny, but she died the day that I received the result from my HIV test. I think Jenny is guilty for this and since that moment Jenny does not exist anymore.

I used to go to Centro Victoria, a rehabilitation centre for drug addicted men, as a volunteer. I liked spending part of my time helping disadvantaged people and supporting them. Two years ago I met Luis, he was attending the centre. I immediately fell in love with him. It was the same for Luis. We were like teenagers looking all day long into each other's eyes.

I started a relationship with him. Soon, after three and a half years, Luis was ready to come out from the centre and to start a new life. We decided to live together. When he left the centre all his belongings filled just one bag: two pairs of pants, one t-shirt and his photo album. We had to start from zero because his family had rejected him a long time ago. He wanted to have everything that he couldn't have before: a family, a job, a normal life; all his friends were dead or in prison and he felt so good because

of our love. But then he started to feel bad, always suffering from stomach problems and thinking it was something he had eaten the day before. He got really thin. He couldn't put on weight even though he ate a lot.

When I got pregnant I discovered I was HIV positive. During the pregnancy I started to feel bad and I kept losing weight. At one point I reached 42 kg. I went to the doctor and he asked for several different tests. On the paper he gave me I read the words "HIV test". It was the first time I thought I could get HIV. I thought it was to do with prostitutes or homosexuals, I swear. I started to cry, I didn't want to go back to the clinic to know the result, it was so scary. So, in the end I went to the clinic with Luis, the doctor told me that I was HIV positive. My head turned, I couldn't stand up and I tried to steady myself on the wall. A few days later Luis discovered he was HIV positive too.

I went to the hospital to give birth through caesarean section. It was horrible, the nurses didn't want to take care of me and nobody touched me because of my condition. When my baby was born a nurse told me: "She'll be like you: sick!" I wanted to die. Finally a doctor came to my bed and explained that we had to wait 18 months to be sure if my daughter was HIV positive or not. Today she is almost one year old. I left my job as a teacher - a job I really liked, because I was pregnant, and I never went back to school. Jenny was a teacher but Jenny is now dead.

So life is hard and I have to find new sources to get money for my little baby like, for example, making scarves or other things made of wool. I attended handcraft workshops organized for women living with HIV, where I learned some skills in order to earn money.

Every morning at 6 o'clock the TV switches on, automatically, on Channel 187. I watch a religious programme until 8 o'clock. The faith in God helps me a lot. When that programme ends, me and Luis have to take our medicine. I put the bottles of medicine close to the TV in order to remind us to take them. Also I put the bottle of milk for my daughter. Since we started the treatment our conditions have been improving every single day. He delivers pizzas in downtown with his motorbike and he comes home late every night. I do all the house work. I can't breastfeed so I have to give her artificial milk. She likes it and she's in a good healthy condition. We have still to wait some more months to know if she's positive or not but I'm sure she's not. I feel it.

When you come out from the MSF clinic with a positive test, someone from the "Self-help group" comes to you and invites you to join the group. This happened to me too. Going to those meetings helped me a lot. It showed me that I was not the only one with this illness and that it is possible to have a normal life even if you have HIV. We chose the name 'Cruzando Fronteras' (Crossing borders) for our group for two reasons. The first one is that if you have HIV you can cross borders and go ahead with your life, doing things, working, meeting friends. The second one is that we want to acknowledge MSF because they helped us in many many ways, not just by giving us pills and treatment.

This testimony was part of a series called "My life with HIV" composed by life testimonies compiled by MSF and published online by the BBC, 1st Dec 2006.

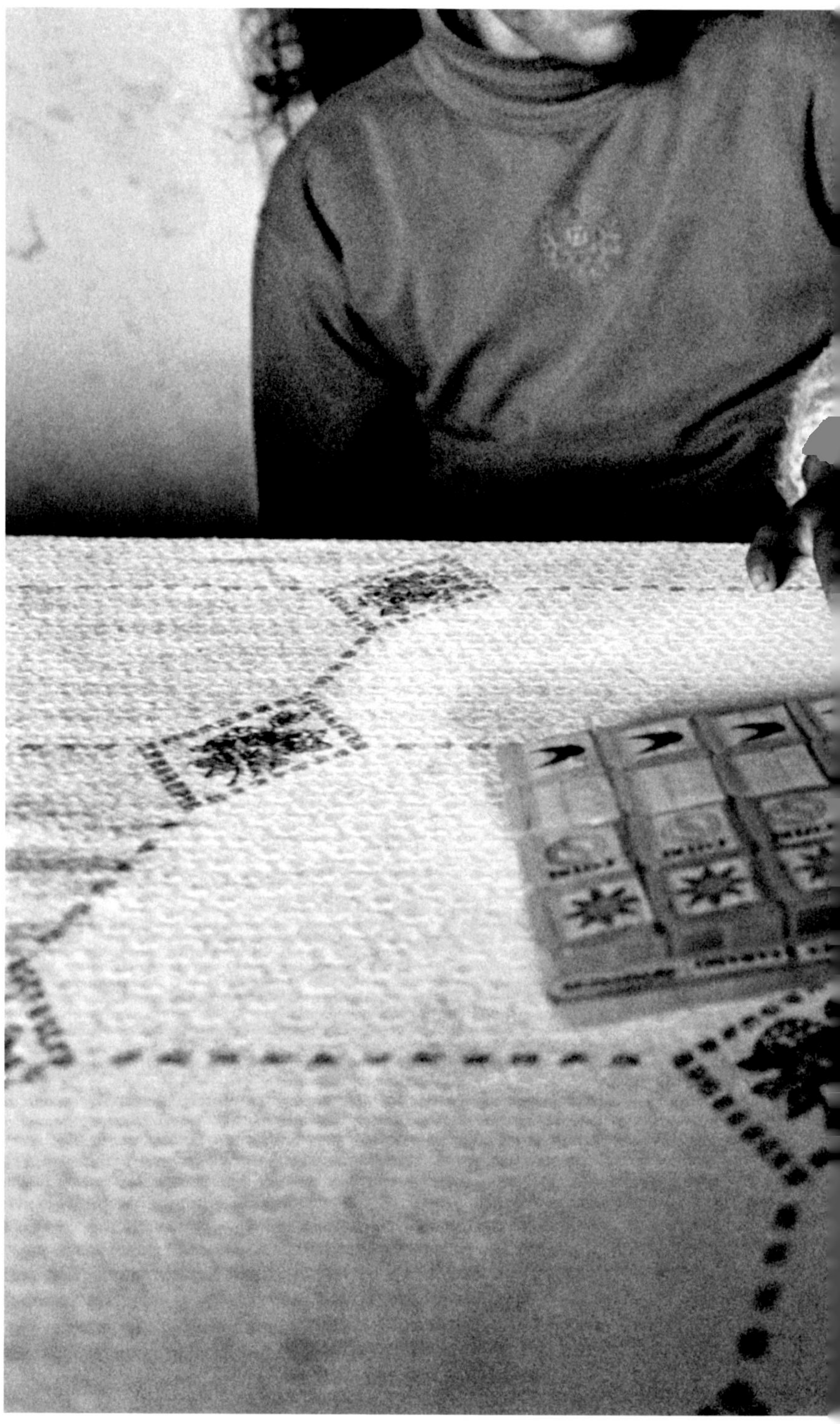

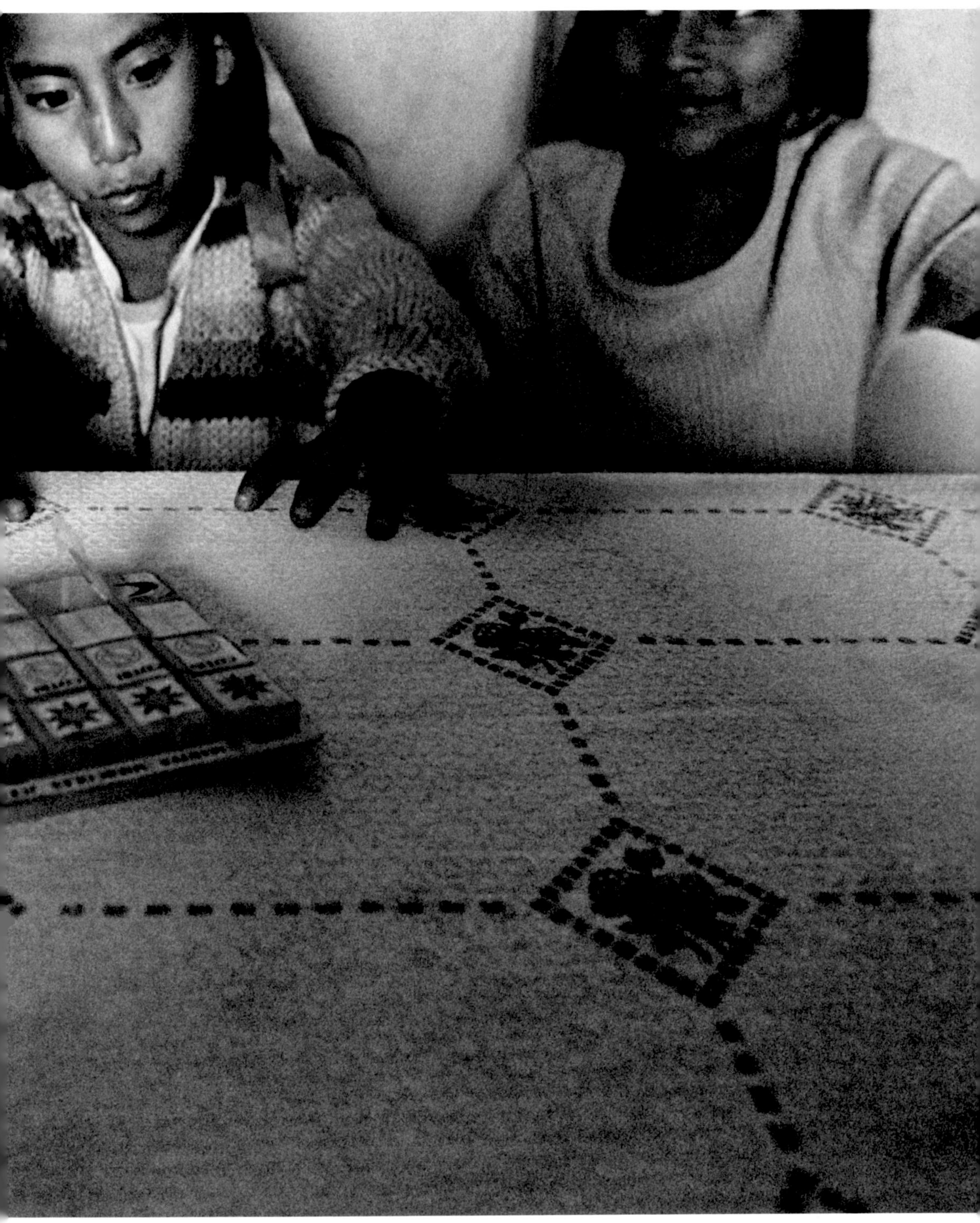

Zoila

My name is Zoila and I am 28 years old. My husband died on 5th March 2004. He had AIDS and he died because of TB. I am HIV positive too. I live in Villa El Salvador with my three children.

I discovered that I was also HIV positive when I was pregnant with my last child, José. When I gave birth to José I didn't believe he could complete one year of life. This is what they told me in the hospital. I started collecting his things. I kept his umbilicus and his newborn bracelet. I kept also the syringe I used during the first weeks to give José his medicine. I had to give him a syrup, which made him so uncomfortable, he used to cry every time, I felt so bad; he was only an infant and he had to take medicine because of me and my illness.

I started writing a diary because I wasn't sure he would survive. That's why, for his first birthday, I bought a huge cake because it was a very special party for us. Now I know José is HIV negative, all because I followed all my prenatal medical checking, got tested and took the treatment without failing.

Someone told me that in town there was a centre where a mother living with HIV could get milk for children. I went out at 7 am to go downtown and look for this centre called San Camilo. I was scared, although I'm from Lima I don't know the city well. I knew I had to do it for my baby. I knocked on the door and went in. The centre was full of mothers living in the centre with their small children. They were all HIV positive and they didn't have any other place to stay. I felt I was not the only mother living with HIV. Compared to them I felt lucky because I had a house for me and my children.

I've got a best friend, Sulema. I was so scared to tell her my diagnosis, I was sure she wouldn't be my friend anymore. But when I told her the truth she held me tight and said, "Don't worry! There are many people living with this illness and they're doing very well. I'm sure everything will be ok." She told me the truth, that she suspected I could have AIDS because of my husband's death and because I was very, very ill at one point, so she did some research on the Internet. She told me that with precautions and medicine my child would be negative. For the first time since I knew my diagnosis I had the hope to have again a normal life. Sulema has been a very important person for me, with her backing I feel I can go ahead.

I have three children. Every birthday of one of my children I can celebrate represents to me a reason for living. They are all my life. The oldest is John Johnson and he's 10 years old. I got pregnant with him when I was only 16 and I had to leave school. Jelin is the only girl, she is the second and wants to become a doctor because, "I don't want to see anymore people sick and suffering like you and dad, I want to take care of sick people." I want to give her more chances, I want her to go to school and have a better life than I have had. And then there is José, who is two years old.

I want to teach my children respect. My husband used to beat me, he drank a lot and he didn't have any respect for me and my body. I want them to live in a different way.

Before I started the treatment I was just lying on my bed all day long. I didn't have enough energy to do anything, I woke up and I started thinking. After the death of my husband I was sure to be the next one to die. I was always thinking: "Today is the last day."

On February 2004 I started to take ARVs. My life changed. A few days afterwards I felt new energies in my body. Before, when I opened my eyes, I only wanted to close them again and keep sleeping all day. Now I wake up, want to do things and have energy to take care of my children, work and walk around.

The ARVs will give me the chance to see my children become older and older and this is the most important thing for me.

One thing I do for a living is to make small jewels with beads: rings, earrings, bracelets, pins, little crowns… I do all these things with my hands. When I work with beads I feel well, I feel realized. One day I want to have a small shop to sell all these pretty things.

I want to earn money and buy something for my children. Our house is empty, we don't have anything. I'd like to buy a radio, I really like music and I love to dance salsa and merengue.

My dream is to buy a TV too. I really like to watch the news on TV. I want to be informed on what's going on in my country, especially regarding health issues, because I know it is absolutely important for my life.

Now I have a boyfriend, his name is Segundo. I met him in a group for people living with HIV supported by MSF. He is a mototaxi driver. He's one of the first who started this job in the barrio. Like many people he had arrived from the province to find a job in Lima.

Before starting the treatment he couldn't work, he had no energy and he was extremely thin. He lives on the 4th floor and at that time he couldn't even come out of his house.

Now he runs on the stairs. My family like him a lot. They see the difference between him and my first husband. Segundo takes care of me. My children like him too. We still do not live together, but one day maybe…

Everybody in my neighborhood (Barrio) knows that I'm HIV positive. I have no fear to say what I am because I want to show everybody that people living with HIV can have a normal life if we get access to medicine. It is so important for us. I've done a psychological test to become a counselor and I passed it. Now I'm attending a course and I know that I'll become a counselor for people living with HIV. I want to learn more about what AIDS means, but also opportunistic infections, ARVs etc. I want to help people like me. Today this is my goal but I know I still have a lot of things to do.

This testimony was part of a series called "My life with HIV" composed by life testimonies compiled by MSF and published online by the BBC, 1st Dec 2006.

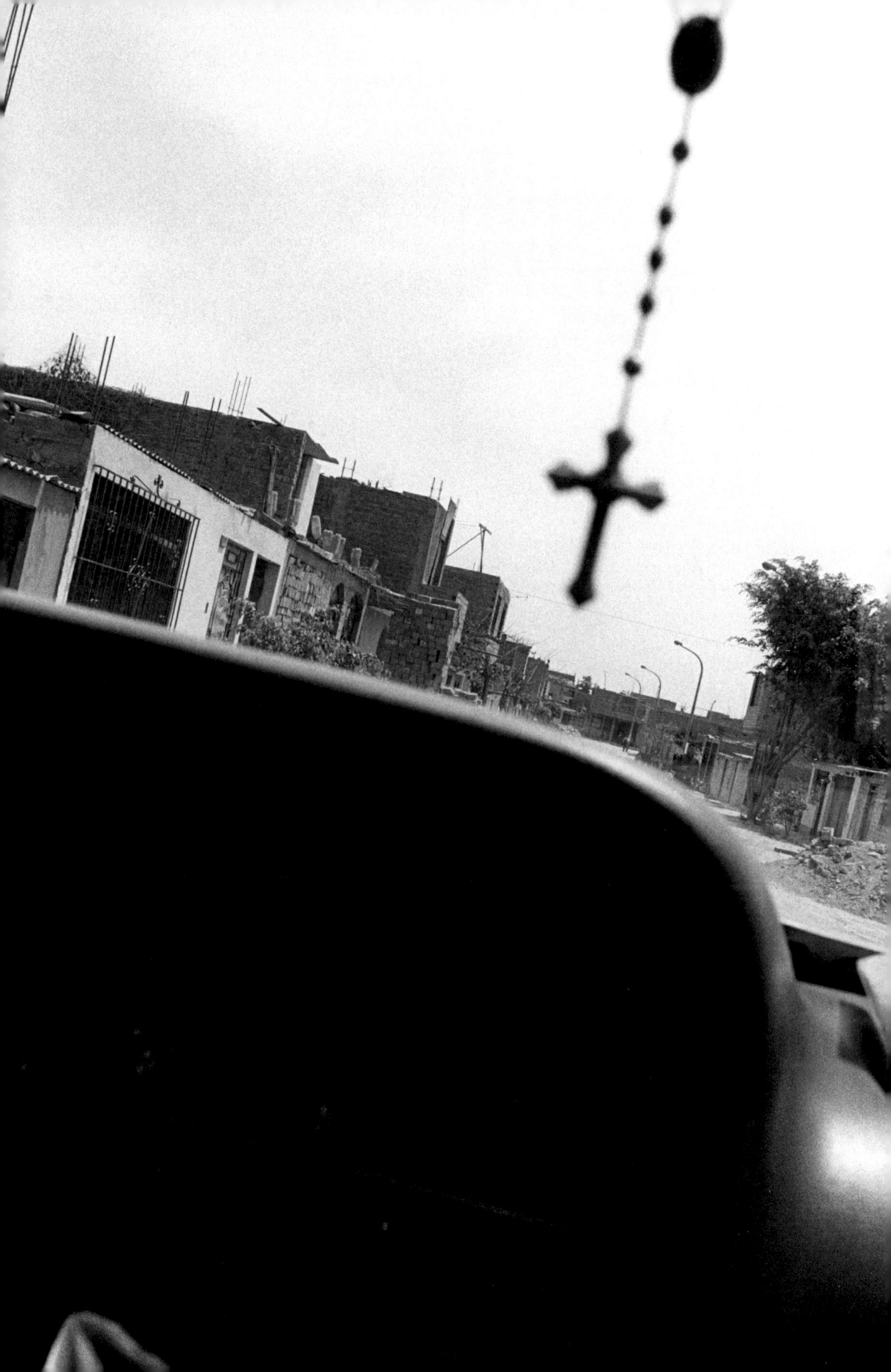

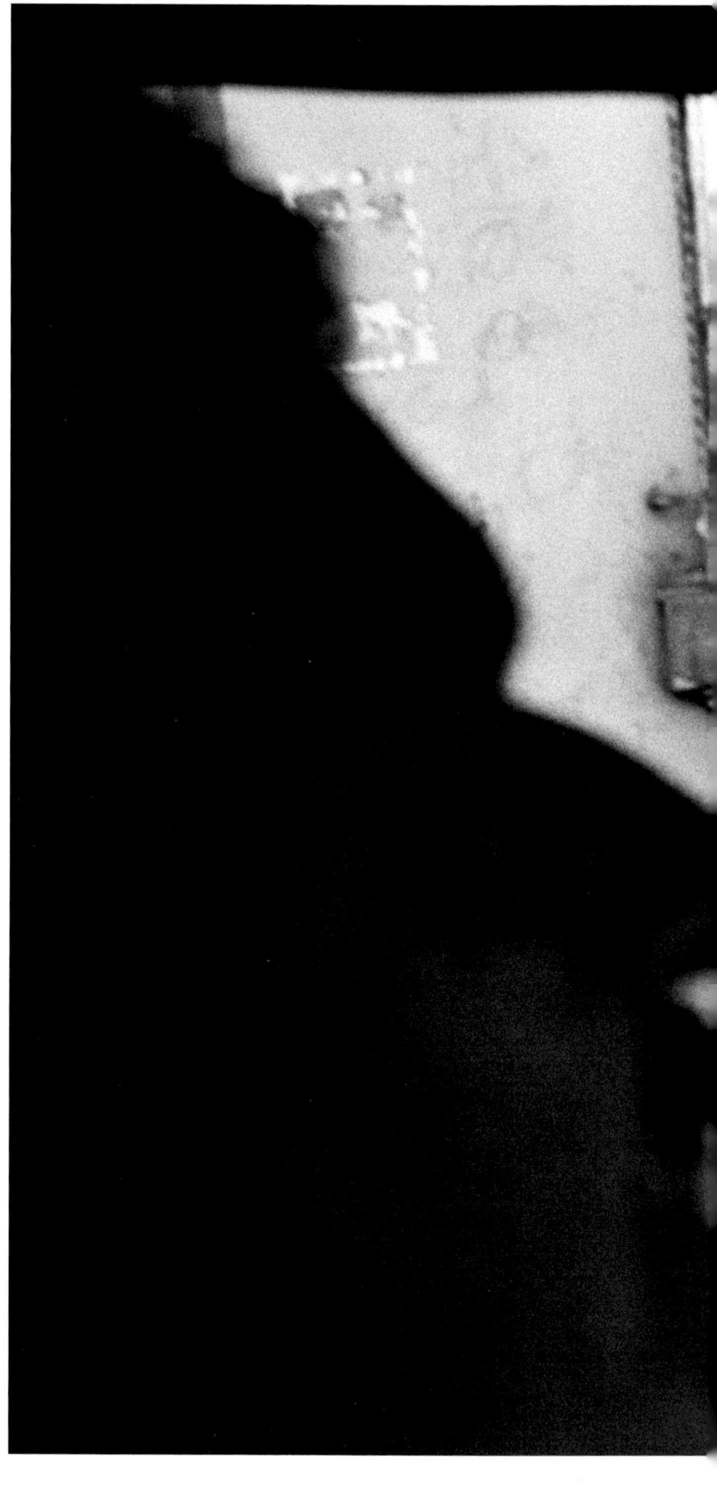

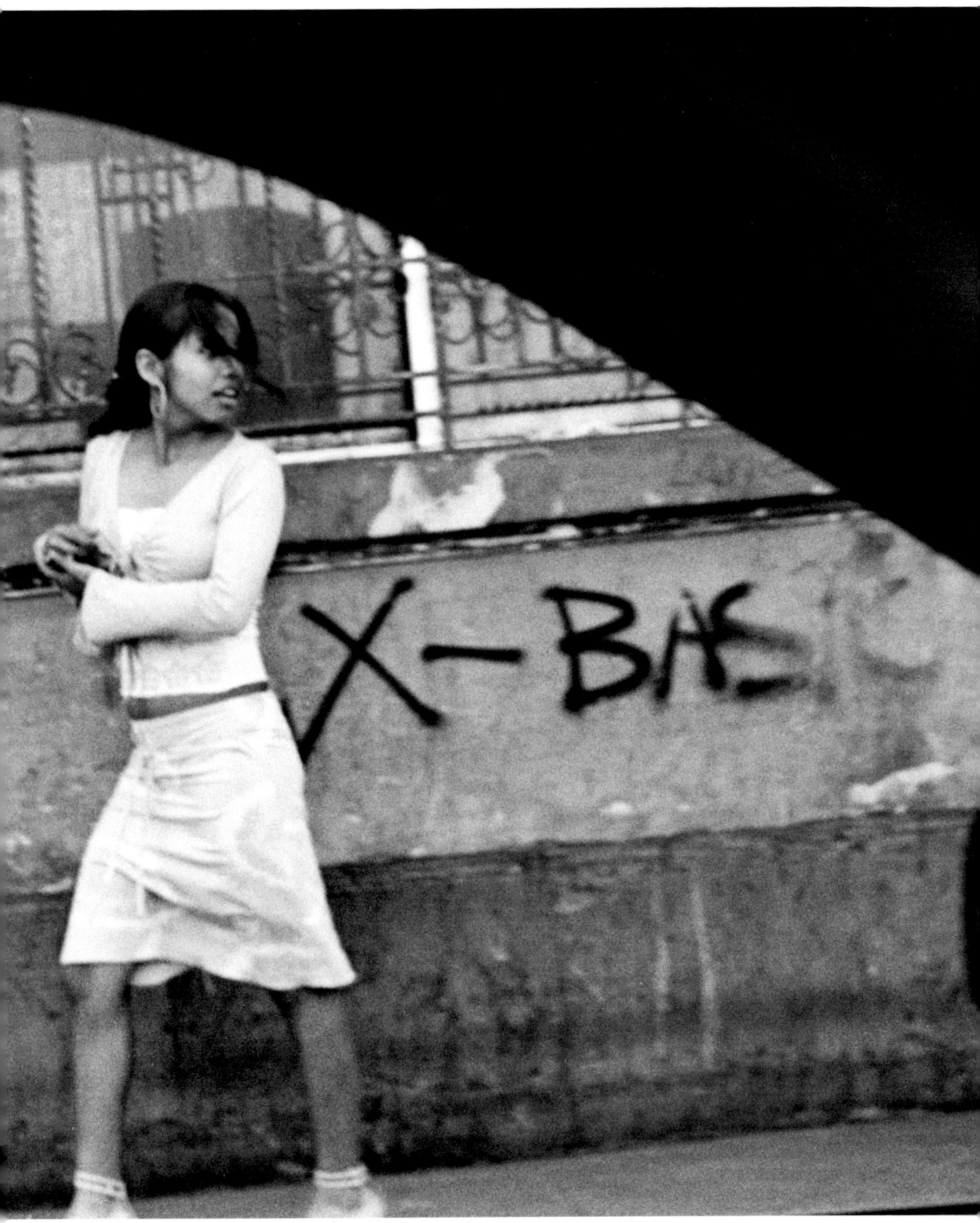
X-BAS

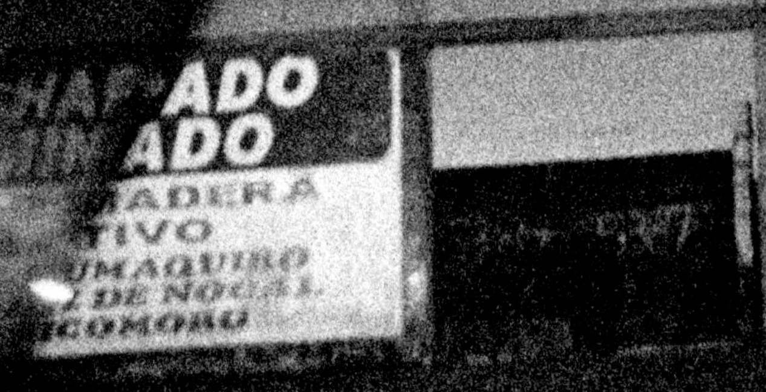
ADO
ADO
ADERA
TIVO
MAQUIN
DE NOCH
COMORO
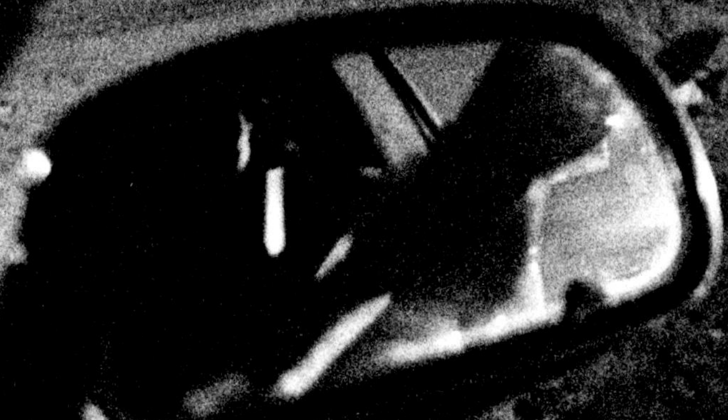

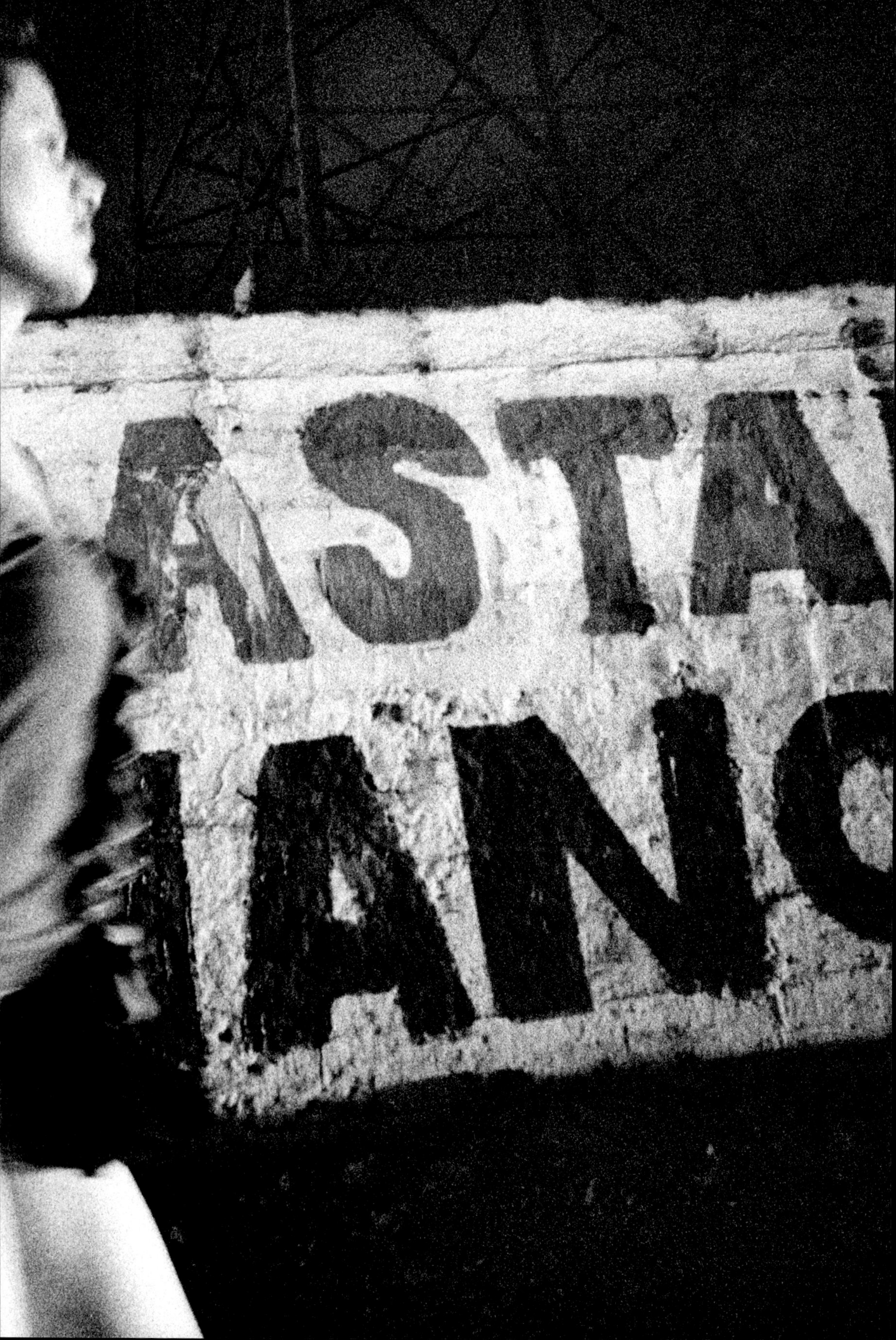
ASTA
TIN

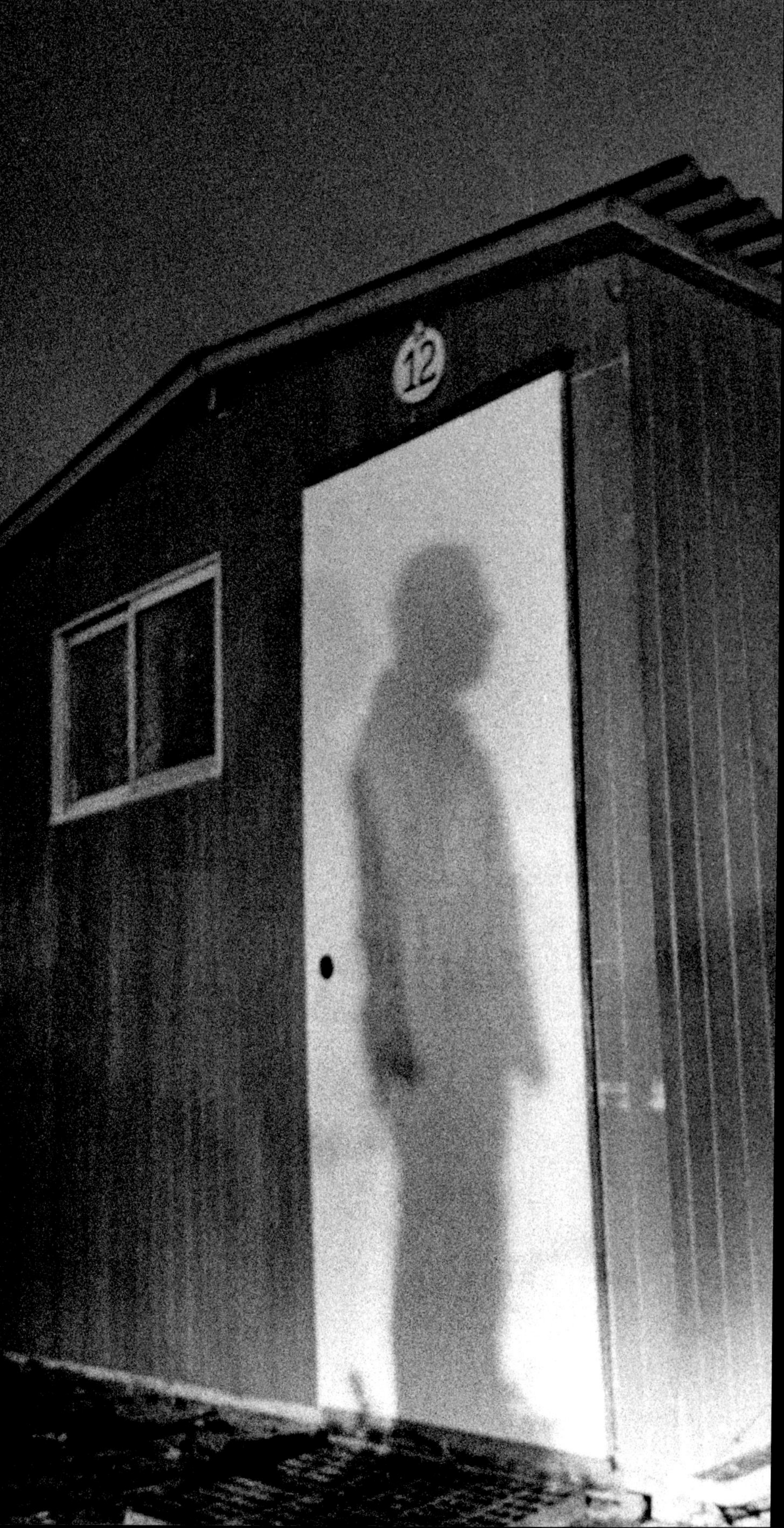

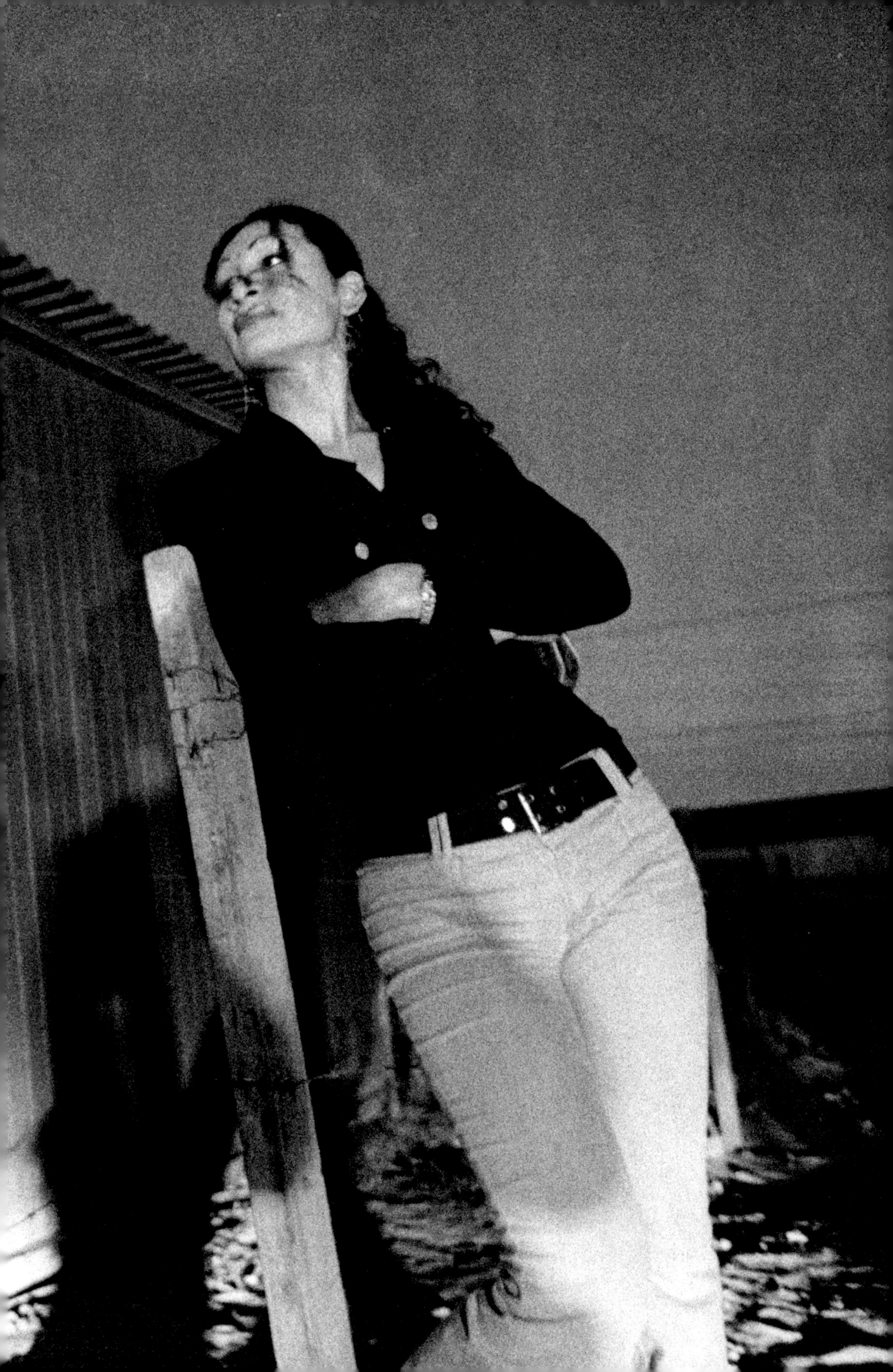

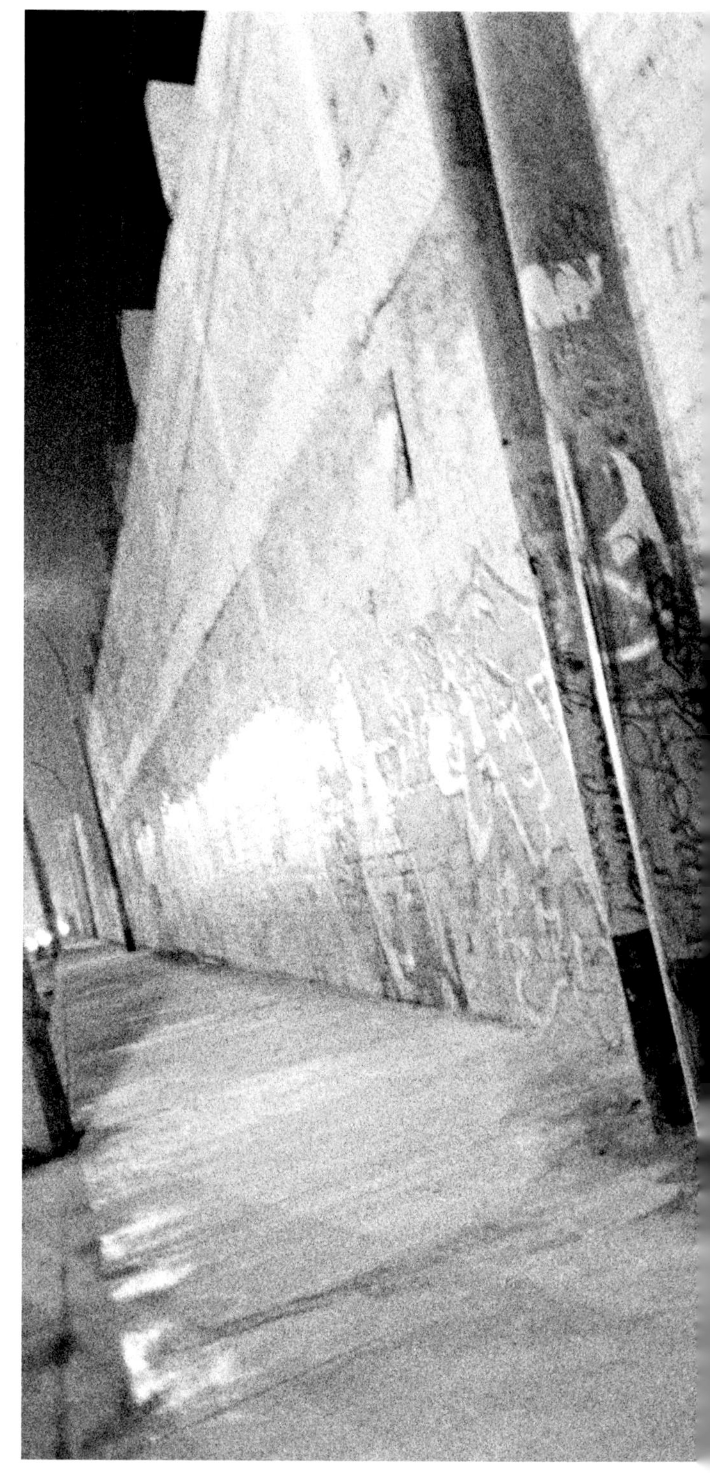

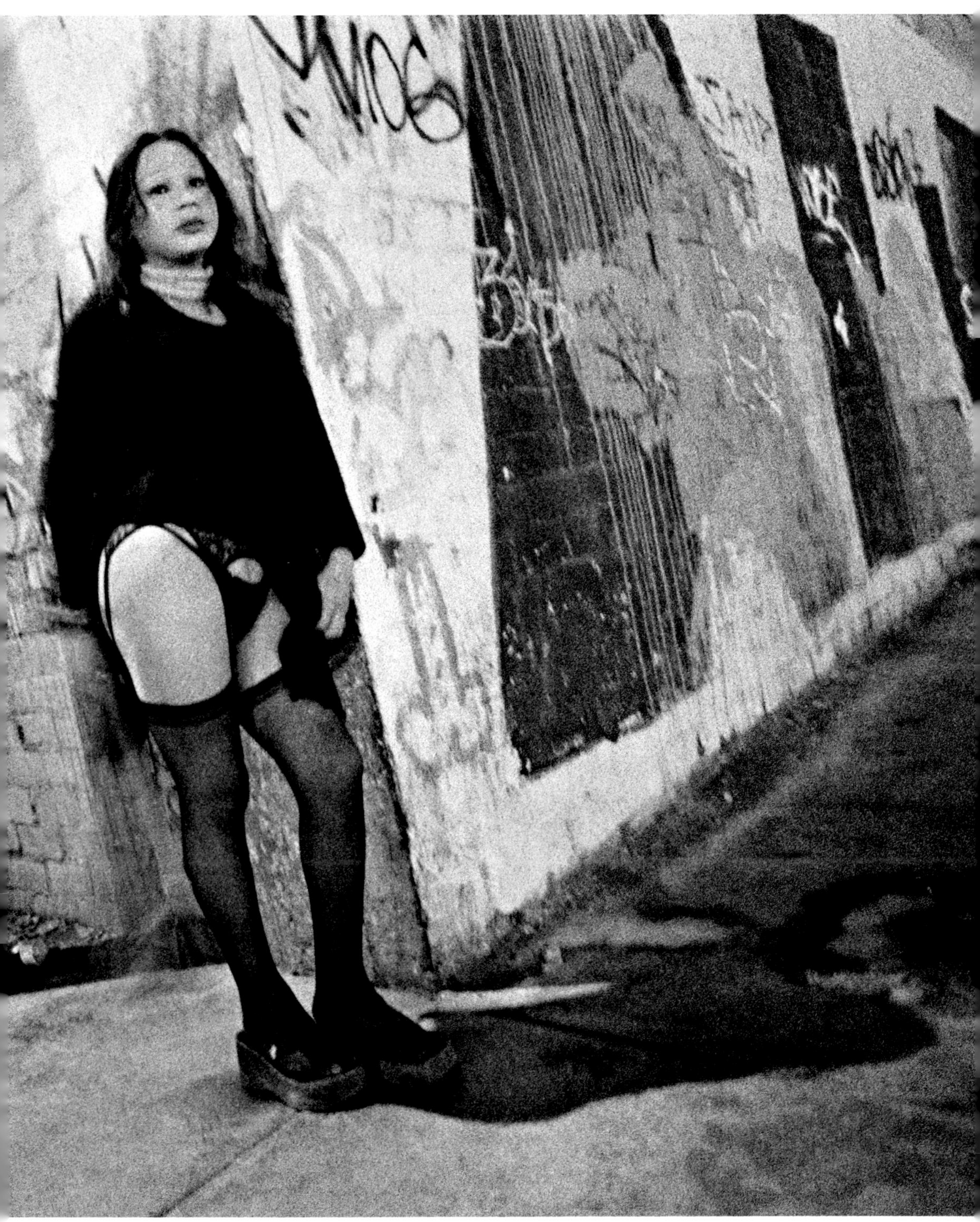

Thalia

20 YEARS OLD · HAIRDRESSER AND SEX WORKER
LIVES ALONE IN VILLA EL SALVADOR

I was a transvestite by the age of 14. I used to wear women's garments and Cleopatra-style make-up, tight pants, wigs and acrylic high heels. I don't care if everybody stares at me, I like to feel free, to be shocking, to flirt with men. They follow me and clown around (term for men who say they are heterosexual, but still have sex with other men). Most of the men in Villa el Salvador do it, in exchange for money if possible. Sometimes, you can see transvestite pechando (when somebody invites you for food or drink or buys you clothes with the intention of having intercourse afterwards) taking care of their points (client for sexual intercourse) with their partners, like flies around them. I only flirt with guys, I cut their hair, ha ha, I give them a smile, I talk to them very softly, I caress them, so they surrender to me.

I love to dance, sometimes at the discos I perform shows impersonating Thalia (a famous Mexican singer, considered a gay icon), that's why everybody calls me "la Thalía". I chose that name for her songs, her voice, her steps. I like her because she is very skinny, even now she is pregnant, she looks great. When I clean the hair salon I always sing her songs and dance like her. All the guys stare at me and I shoot them a look because I want them to respect me. If you are a queer you have to have a lot of nerve, otherwise you are done for.

I ran away when I was 14 years old. I used to live in Callao. My dad knew that I was gay and he hit me, "Hit me once more and I'll run away" I used to say. And my father saw me leaving with my little box to Rogelio's house, a queer that used to live at the other corner of the street. She helped me, I cooked for her, did the laundry, and thanks to her I learned how to be a hairdresser and I helped her in her salon. She used to tell me, "Men have to support you, why should we pay for them?"

While living with her I myself started as a sex worker. At night I dealt with cars (sex work on the street), and I made up to 50 soles ($16 USD) in one day so I started paying for my own things. As I worked late at night, sometimes had to sleep under a bridge, covering myself with sheets of cardboard, very thin ones; there I slept, feeling very cold, next to drug addicts. I had to be very alert to avoid them doing me any harm, I used to carry a broken bottle as a weapon if they went too far with me. I can tolerate if they insult me, but I can't tolerate that they touch me. If you touch me I will destroy you.

Then I moved to La Victoria, to an alley. By that time I had joined Projoven (Program of the Ministry of Labor offering technical training to teenagers and young men in various areas to help them to find a job) where I learned a lot and worked in a hairdressers. I kept on doing sex work, but now only with older men.

And so I ended up in Villa el Salvador. I rented a small room, and there I live. My grandmother and my aunt live close to me, but I don't want to live with them because I have small nephews and nieces and I care about what they may say... since I am like this. So I manage to live by myself, I am already 20 years old. Here I work in a hairdresser's and also do sex work.

I adore working at the hairdressers; my dream is to have one myself, but it's hard... At the hairdressers I make little money; I receive a percentage, so I have to work on the streets in order to get some extra cash to buy my stuff for my future hairdressers.

Working on the streets is hard work, I get there at 8.30pm and stay until 2am, and do that Monday, Tuesday, Wednesday, Friday, Saturday and Sunday. With the clients, you have to do it in an abandoned construction site, in the dark, in an alley, behind the bushes. There we do well you know...that alley is used as a hotel. How much do we charge? 6 soles ($2 USD). In one night I can make 10 soles ($3.20 USD), 15 soles ($4.80 USD), 20 soles ($6.30 USD). It depends on how good you look and the weather. If it is a cold day or rainy, it's worse. Even us, we want to go home! On weekends you can make more money.

Now with such cold weather, I wear pants, very warm. I am not too uncovered, but I still have success. I also have clients that call my cell phone. I am thinking of putting pictures of myself on the Internet, having sex, to do racket and to promote myself overseas! I have been asked to travel to Argentina, to work on the streets, but I'm not that bold, I am a bit afraid, I don't know why but I feel that traveling is not a good idea, everything is going to be wrong.

Working on the streets is very risky, they throw stones at you from cars, they spit at you; rowdy guys come and you have to hide from them. When the Serenazgo (Municipal Security Service) come we all get our high heels off and we run no matter where. They rob you! Once, they caught me, but they didn't do anything to me; they released me the next morning at 6am. Many transvestites have been killed on the streets, and there are still some killings. Some men hate us, they're homophobic. That's why I check up and don't stay out too late at night, because it is too dangerous...

Competition among us is very hard, it's not easy to get clients. The one who has boobs wants to destroy the one who hasn't. I don't have them but I am good looking, I show my legs, I stand on the side of those who have boobs and I wear miniskirts, showing my legs, because the one who has boobs doesn't have good legs. Men feel attracted to me. That's why an envious queer once cut my face with a broken bottle. I saw my blood running down my face, I felt very nervous, like crazy, I lost control, attacked and almost killed that crazy queer with my own hands.

In general, most transvestites do not use condoms, mostly the younger ones, because they have a man who tells them he is faithful. Men fool you, they tell you things like, "you are as pretty as a rose," and you believe them. Men are very clever, but they don't like to use condoms. I started having sex when I was 11, and until I was 14 I made it bald (without a condom), I was so naïve! Now I have medical checks every month in San Jose[1] and every two months I am tested. The care is good, doctors are very patient with us... They examine us, take our pants off, and I say, "Doctor, don't touch my vagina" and he turns very serious, ha, ha. I am lucky I don't have HIV, because I'm very careful.

I have had friends that died from HIV, like La Gaviota. She was a doll, with blonde hair. That's why to the younger ones I tell them to be careful, men may tell you, "you are pretty", but use a condom, because HIV is everywhere.

There is no ideal partner, all men always try to get money from you. With me it's hard, I have been with 35 men because of my body, and not one of them has ever taken any money from me. I would probably accept a well-educated guy, with good character to be with me, then I would get used to it. You cook, do the laundry, and then men get used to being with you. But if I have the slightest doubt or anybody tells me that he/she has seen my partner with another queer, I would tell him, "If you are with a queer, forget about me". There are thousands of Thalias, but no one like me; I am a hairdresser, but I'm not stupid. I'll grab your stuff and throw it away, I won't wait for you to do it. If you want to live with a gay you have to think it over, because I am not a woman, I have the same as you, but I am more woman than you.

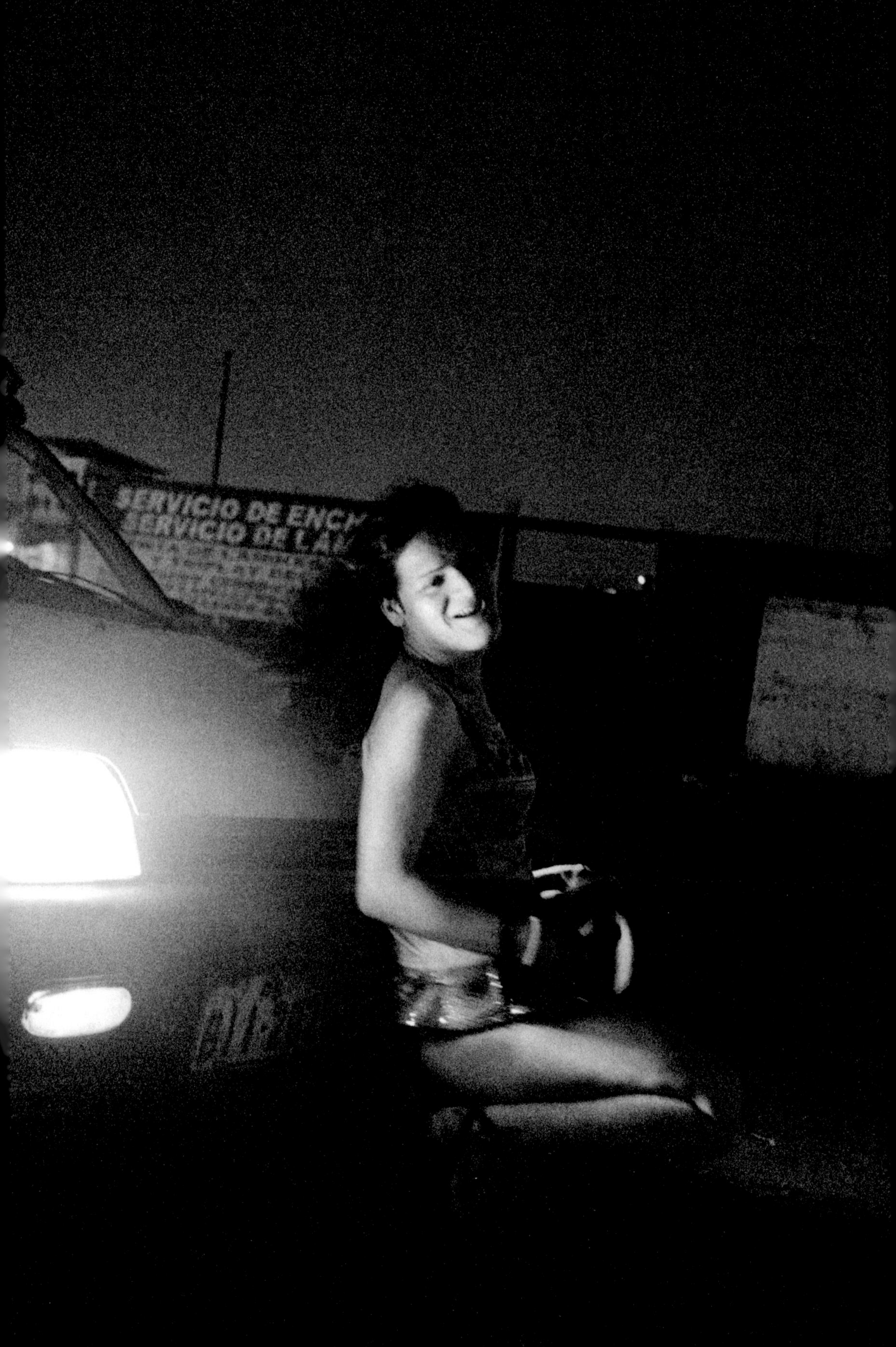
SERVICIO DE ENC
SERVICIO DE LA

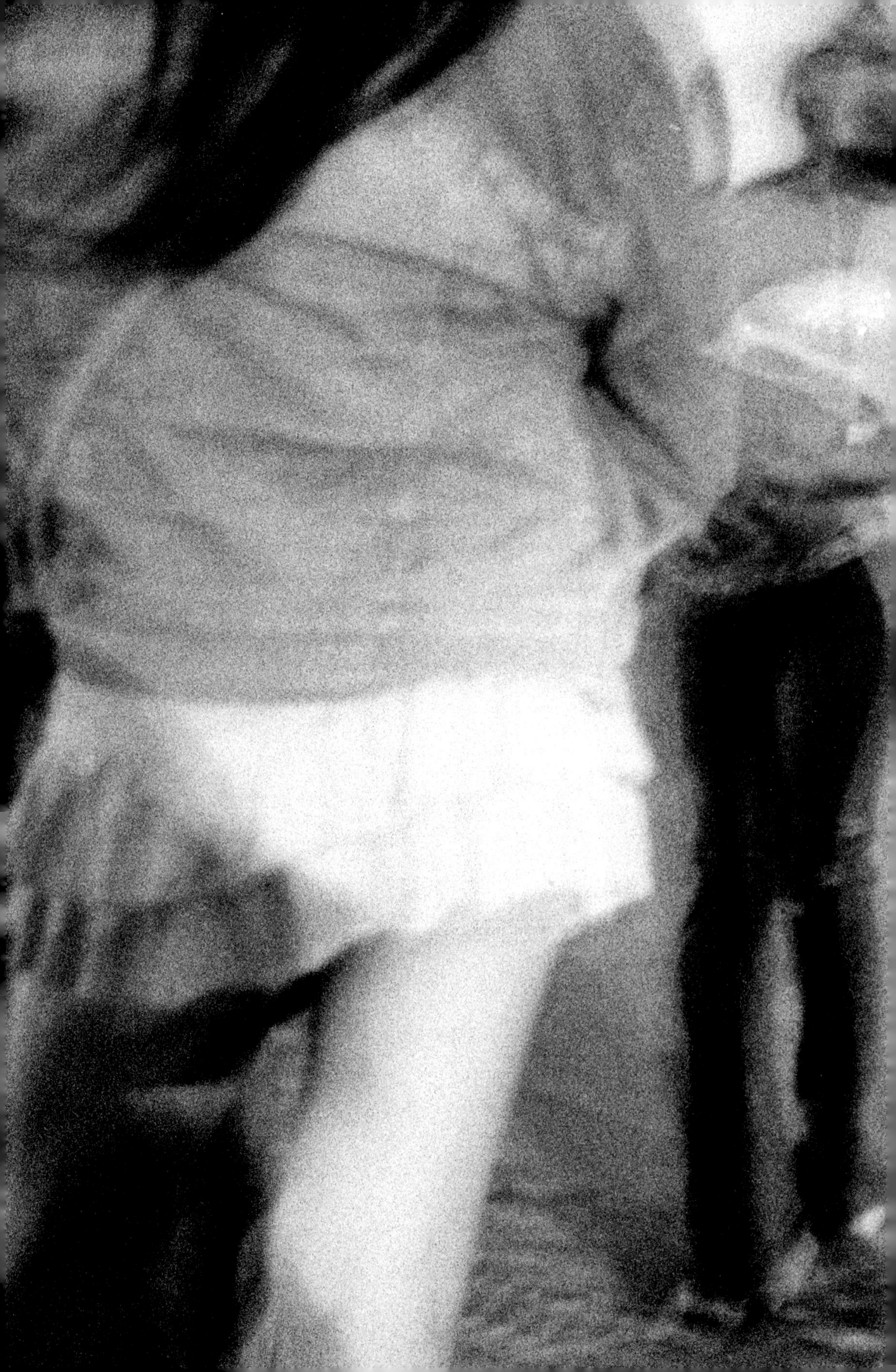

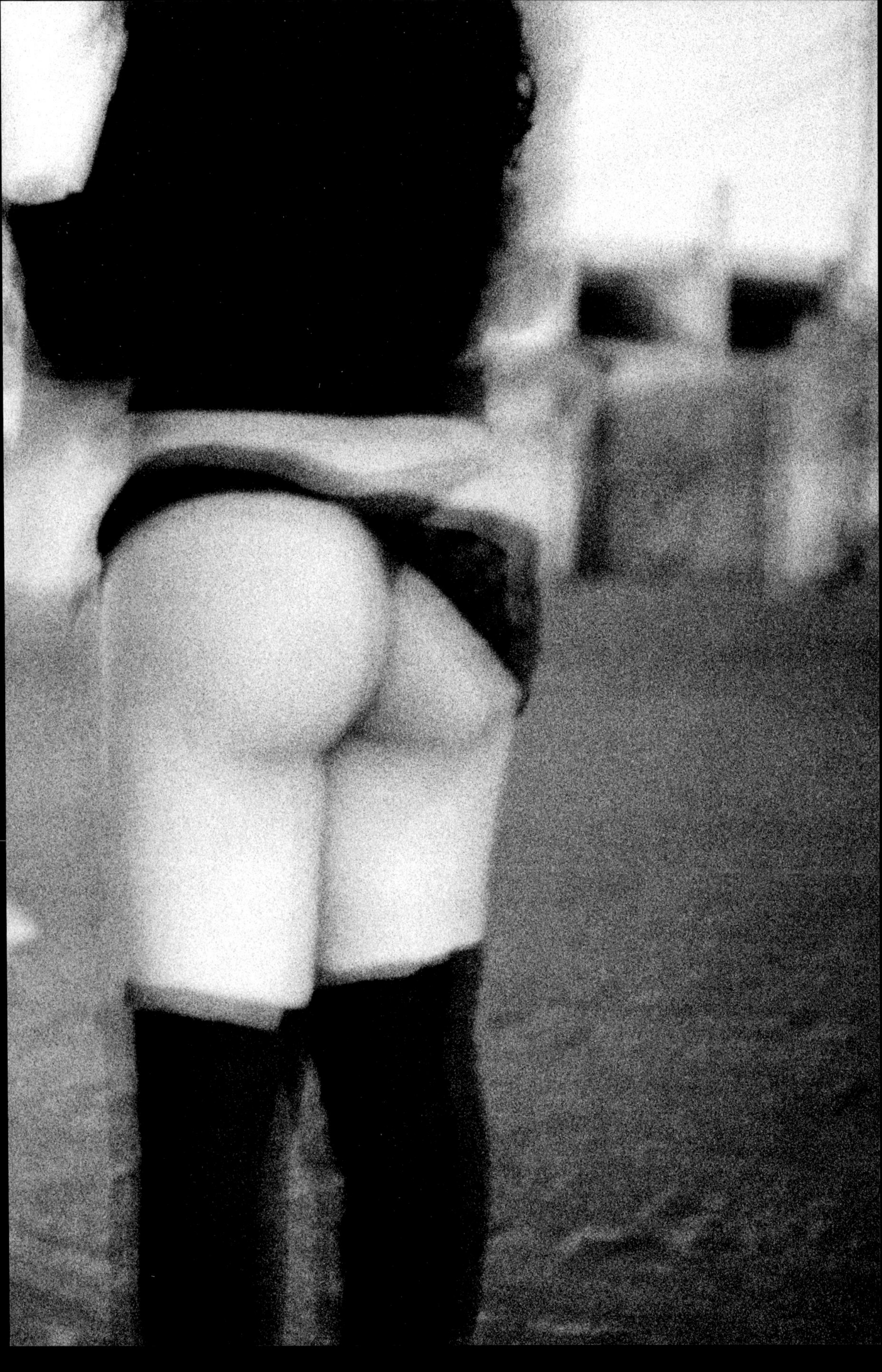

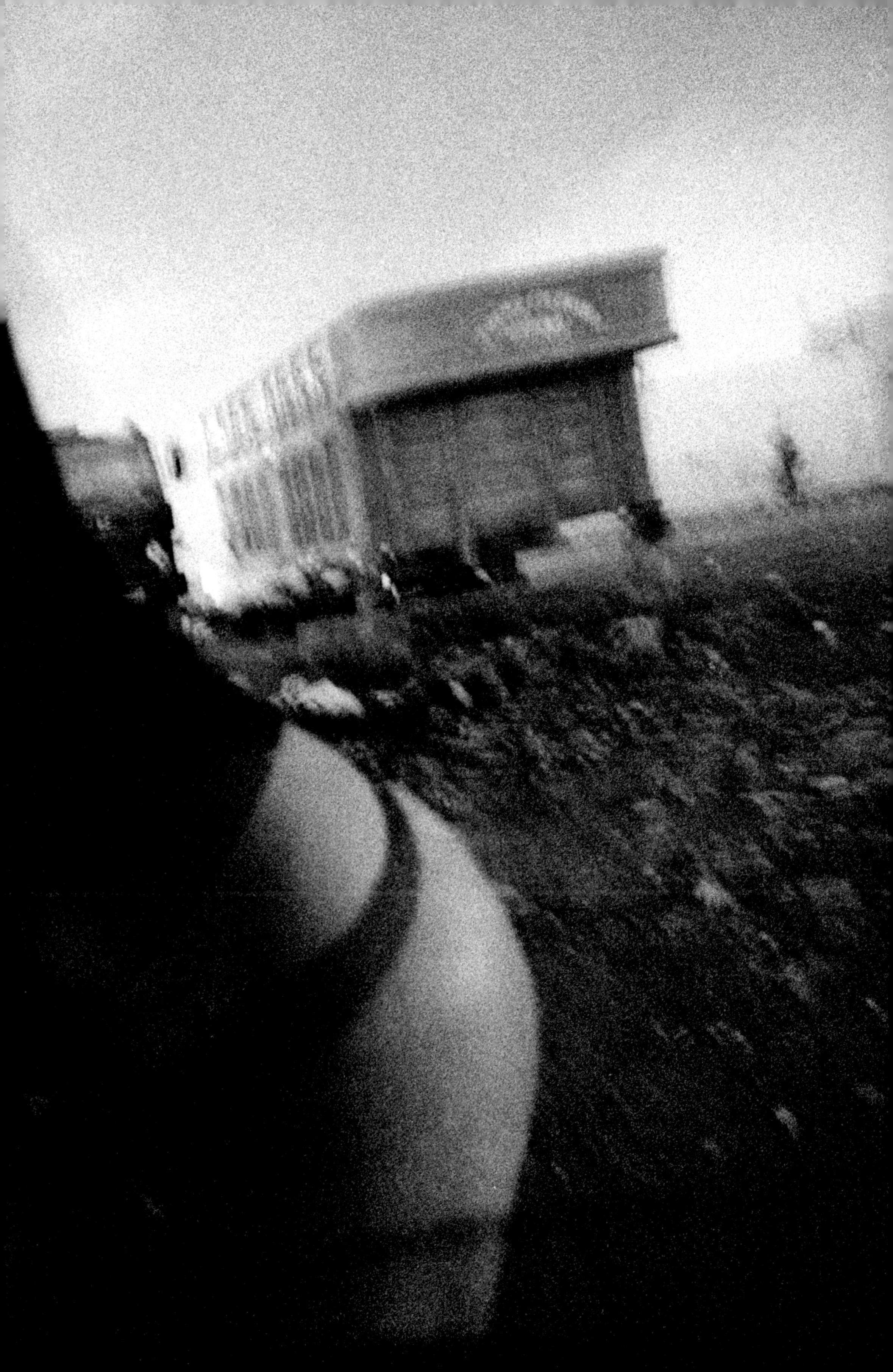

Martina

41 YEARS OLD · HAIRDRESSER AND SEX WORKER
LIVES IN VILLA EL SALVADOR WITH HER PARENTS

I entered Universidad de San Marcos because I wanted to study Psychology. But I wanted to change…. How was I going to become a psychologist with long hair and female breasts? That was the reason I quit school…

I was under treatment for many years to "become a male", if you know what I mean. My father used to sell food in a kiosk at the Mental Health Hospital and since I was a child, I used to play in the backyard. All the doctors saw the way I walked. It wasn't a boy's walk, it was too girlish. They opened a medical record for me and I started a treatment that lasted for many years. But it didn't work. I received male hormones and nothing happened. I was even locked up with a girl in a room so that I could, you know… ha, ha. They gave me something to make me feel sleepy, but my reaction was to hit the girl.

As they couldn't change me, they talked to my dad and my mom to turn me into a woman. They said I should get a partner so I wouldn't go out and get sick, because I used to run away a lot looking for men. My mother accepted it: she has always supported me. I attended two sessions to receive hormones in order to have a woman's life, but I quit because the hospital was too far away and appointments took a very long time, they talked to me for hours, and I would get bored. If I had accepted, things would now be different. My whole body would have been more feminine. As a kid I wanted to be a queer, very stunning, as they say, you know? Blonde, tall, with lots of silicone… I wanted to be an actress or a singer.

In my last year of high school I used to skip classes and I drank a lot. I used to go to places where boys used to get high and have sex. I wanted to have sex with a man and I was with four, five, or six… one wasn't enough!

I went to the streets looking for money. When I started, at age 16, it was OK, I was very successful. I got there at 10pm. and I stood there. There were 4 of us in one block, each one with her own space. We used to get high because we were cold and we were using miniskirts, with cleavages, almost naked. We worked until 5 or 6 in the morning. Then I had a warm soup or the whole group went to have some drinks. I would get home around 6am.

Since my dad was always drunk, he didn't notice, and as I used to sleep in a separate room, even my mother didn't notice anything.

As they say, every queer has their own way to get along. Well, I guess they sensed something. At 8am I would rush to school where I used to be very sleepy, sometimes my face wasn't clean enough, although I tried to remove the make-up, some color would stay on my face. That's why I was called a "queer" at school, and they made fun of me.

We used to get dressed in a hairdressers where we had our dresses. There I disguised myself. I say "disguise" because when I was a teenager, getting fake boobs and stuffing your body was actually "disguising". The queers atthe hairdressers gave me the fake boobs to wear, they were really old queers and what they couldn't wear anymore, they gave to all of us, the beginners. When I started to make my own money I started buying my own stuff: clothes, accessories, I loved my boots.

At the beginning I had problems with some queers, but I had my godmother to protect me. When she took me there for the first time, she told them: "She is my daughter" so nobody would harm me. Her name was the Shazam. But she passed away.

In the streets I met a lot of friends, some had undergone surgery or had traveled to Italy. They told me to go with them, but as I wanted to have a lover and I felt sad for my mother, I stayed. In addition, I never saved money, I drank it. Now, as the police are after us, the youngsters want to go away to other countries and most of them come back transformed, operated. They save their money and spend it all on small surgeries, so they will have more clients, and so on. Those who travel, lend money to their friends so that they can build their bodies. These friends travel afterwards, and they have to work hard to give that money back. Over there they earn more and can pay their debts sooner. Some of them even manage to buy a four-storey house and cars.

Working on the streets is very hard. It's very cold out there and the cops themselves steal your money. You have to hire piranhas (children and teenagers living alone on the streets and dedicated mostly to crime activities for survival) to take care of you, otherwise they will rob you or will rob your clients.

Generally, we have intercourse in various construction areas, on the side of the street, because we get so little money. If we get paid better, we go to a hotel. But for 10 soles ($3.20 USD) just there, in the streets. It's quicker there. We do penetration mostly, but some guys want a blow jack and penetration. Then we charge 20 soles ($6.30 USD). Of course, if you do chichi (when the sex worker mugs wallets or watches from their clients) you can get more money. The client concentrates himself on kissing you, sucking your boobs and you work with your fingers.

They call us older ones 'grannies'. They call me that with all respect because I am old and I know everything. I used to be a brat. I have used bottles, knives, I was a fighter and I got known as that. And I have my protégés: Coneja, Candy and Rata. Now I only work in the discos of Los Laureles and Piedra de Papa, but there is a lot of competition there. I don't work on the street anymore because I'm old and it's too cold, and my defenses are low. I only go to the street when I need money. In a good night I could make 50 soles ($16 USD), otherwise I get just enough for my bus ticket, 5 soles ($1.5USD).

At the hairdresser salon I earn a percentage. Some days I make 6 soles ($2 USD), others 20 ($6.30 USD), then I compensate. But it is not enough because I have to pay for electricity, food, water, telephone and get my stuff. That's why I have to work on the street to compensate. My dad still works in his kiosk, and my sister works too.

I always have had my partner, since the doctors told my mom that I had to have him. That's why they built me my own room. I have had partners that have lived in my house and I have had lovers in the streets. It's better to have your partner at home, because you can see him all the time, you sleep with him, you wake up with him and you do things together. It's different. I turned more home-loving. I didn't want to have another man because I had one at home. I met my partners at the bar or on the streets. They were clients. They liked the way I was. Two of them were shot dead by street fighters while watching over me when I was working.

My partners aren't homosexuals, they are men. I have had lovers that act as men on the streets, but when we are alone, they want to hold my dick and I don't like that. My partners have to be very male.

I have been two years under ARV treatment, and everything is going well. I was really sick and if it were not for the antiretroviral (ARV) I wouldn't be here. More than ten years ago, the queer that runs the hairdressers where we used to dress passed away, and then all the other queers started to die, one after the other. Everybody said to me: "And you, why haven't you died too if you have had sex with the same guys?" Maybe because I never paid attention to that, I have lived a normal life, and never been particularly depressed.

In 2001, I went to San José Clinic for my condoms to work on the street, and just out of curiosity I asked to be tested, and I turned out to be positive. I said to myself, "If death takes me away, it's OK," because I was sick of going to the hospital and having tests. I lost a lot of weight and when I reached 47kg I knew I had to make an appointment. I saw the MSF containers, and the doctor told me: "Here they will test your CD4, they will give you everything," as normally, having a CD4 was very expensive (you have to pay 150 soles ($47,6 USD) and I was not able to access it, because I had no money, not even for food.

The treatment has changed my life; it has helped me to acknowledge that I'm a human being. Before, being a healthy person, I never wanted anything. But now I have recovered myself, I went back to work, I stopped drinking,

I even paid for my things. The treatment raised my self-esteem.

As soon as MSF leaves - because that's something foreseen - what will happen with the drugs? The way the hospital's workers treat us is not the same as the doctors'.

Five to ten years from now I will be the same... my goal is to keep on working, stop drinking and as for the life I used to live, that's history... I have changed too much. The former Martina was a drunk, he used to have sex with three, four men on a daily basis. Nowadays, I don't drink, I'm more responsible, I think about saving money, what I'm going to eat or what I have to pay for. Right now my goal is to pay for the hairdressers that I want to get, it will be transferred to me, I've got a loan from the bank, I have to save money. As soon as I get it, I will name it "Martina", because I am well known as "la Martina". There she comes, granny "la Martina" everybody says.

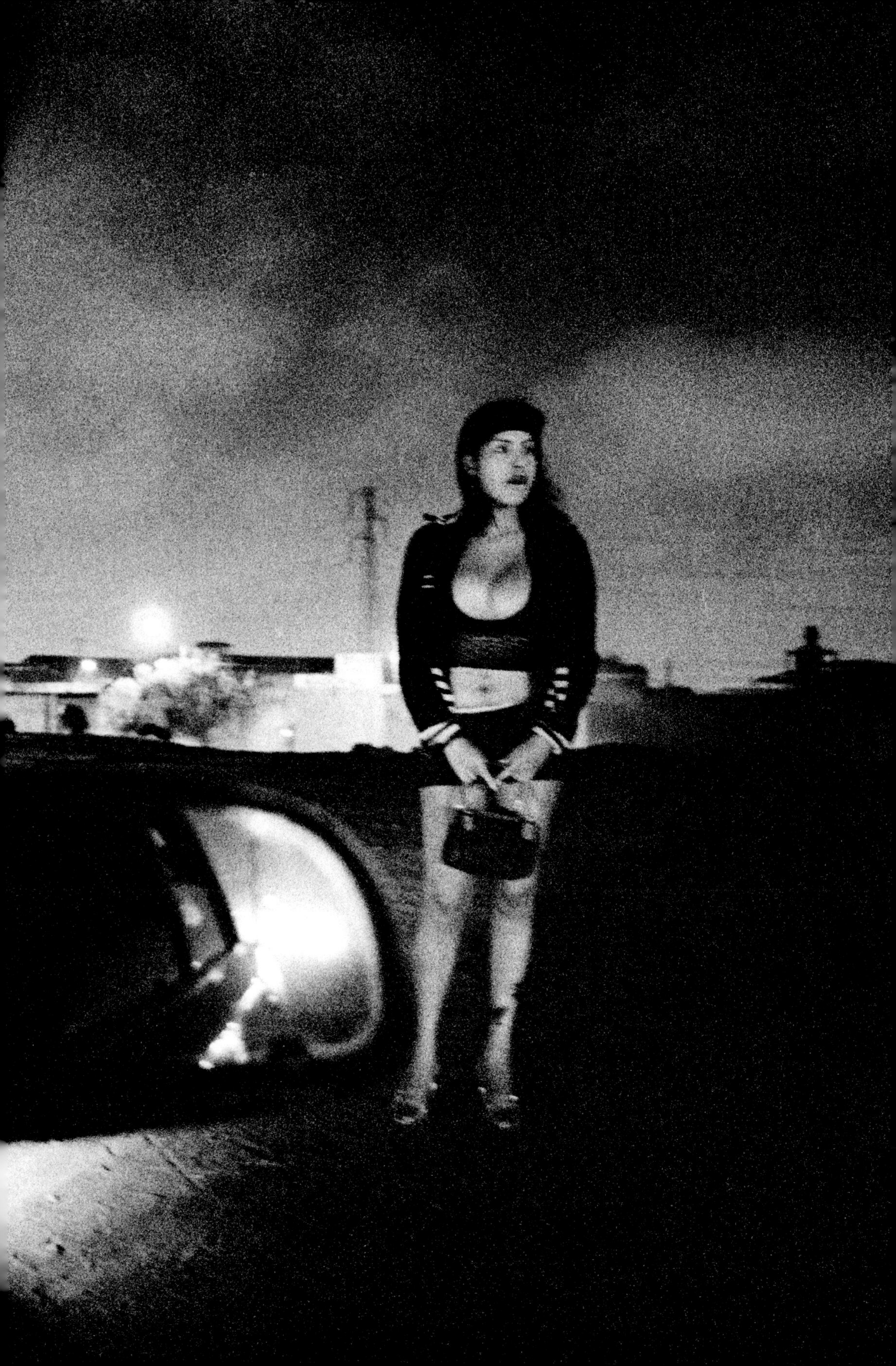

ROSA

45 YEARS OLD • HOUSEWIFE AND SEX WORKER
HAS AN ADULT SON • LIVES IN CALLAO WITH HIM AND HER DAUGHTER-IN-LAW

I have been working for 17 years. Sometimes I work in hotels, my friends (customers) call me in the morning and we arrange to meet.

Needless to say, we were very poor. I had my first boyfriend when I was 13 and at 14, I became pregnant. We were forced to get married but that marriage went up in smoke because we were kids. He was 17.

I remember when I was 28, when I was working in a factory, a workmate asked me if I wanted to work. I got mad: "Are you crazy, me working as a whore?" But with a teenage son and a miserable salary, I thought it was worth it. The first day I cried desperately behind the door... but I went ahead, what the heck. Some of the customers were the ones who put me at ease. Some understand very well... they teach you how to work, and the sex poses. The other girls don't teach you anything! On the contrary, if you're new, they become envious. They leave you to suffer.

I work 6 days a week. I lead a quiet life at home and work from 4 to 10 at night. On weekends, I have more patrons (regular customers). My service is complete, that is a blow jack and posing, it costs 20 soles ($6.30 USD); if they want more time or some fantasies I charge more, 100 soles ($31.80 USD). We pay 20 soles ($6.30 USD) for a room, bed and two rolls of toilet paper for those 6 hours; it doesn't matter if we have 1 or 10 customers. We rent the fluorescent lamps and mirrors. The customer pays 13 soles ($4.10 USD) as an entry fee and pays for the service. Each girl decorates her own room and fixes her bed as she pleases, she can even put a rug out on the floor if she wants.

Once something terrible happened to me, because there, they really take care of us. It was in a massage salon. We were alone and about to close when a customer walks in and points at us with a gun. I remember and I shiver. He made the manager tie up the 10 girls that were there. He pointed the gun at my head! It was madness, we cried and begged. He raped two friends, he couldn't rape me because I was squeezing my legs very hard because I wanted to pee. He stole our money,our the radios, he put everything he could in his bag and left. Shaking, we called the police but they never caught him. I thought I was going to die.

We have checkups every 28 days, at the health center and we have the ELISA test every six months.

If we are healthy, they stamp our cards and we can continue working. If you have a STI (Sexually Transmitted Infection) or HIV they don't give you the card. The girls that come out positive have to work in the street, they are not controlled there. But let me tell you they must be very few because here we always use condoms, even though we don't get them from the health center anymore, we still have to buy them or the customer brings them. Now it is a law, your little condom. Even so, there are customers who offer more money, 100 soles ($31.80 USD), to do it without a condom, and there are some girls who accept. I tell them: "Is that what your life is worth? 100 soles?" And they get mad at me and ask me why I mess with their lives. Here there are ladies, almost old women, who continue working, they say they will die as they lived. I will retire in a couple of years because when I am standing in front of the door of my room waiting for the customers, I think, "What am I doing here?" But let me tell you, you get accustomed to easy money. That is to say, here, you always have work and you earn money. It is easy to get into this business but it is hard to get out. At 45, where am I going to get a job? But let me tell you one thing, it is not as productive as before especially with all those new young girls.

I have worked very hard as a sex worker and I have withstood many things to make a living, build my house, support my son and give him a profession; now he manages a dance salon. He is 29 years old. I live with him and his wife. If I told him what I did, I am sure he wouldn't forgive me, and he wouldn't want to see me anymore. When we are watching TV and the news talks about how a brothel has been raided, he foul-talks about the girls and I feel bad: "If you only knew I have been doing the same things for years, and I go through the same things these girls do. If you only knew that with this kind of job you were able to finish school and register at the institute." That is why I don't dare tell him, or my sisters, whom I get along well with but who would slam the door in my face if they knew, for all that about decency and morality.

I don't know why my son doesn't realize what I do. He and his wife are usually out after noon and come back at midnight. I leave in the afternoon and always try to be back by at least 10pm. What I do is buy women's clothes, accessories, purses and makeup to let them believe I sell those things, that I have customers all over Callao. The truth is I do sell some things to the other girls when there is time. I have to be some kind of magician with my family to keep my secret, I have to remember what I have said, and take care when I speak to my customers over the phone so they don't know I am talking to customers but to possible buyers. It is crazy, that is why I want to retire.

When I retire, well, I have some savings. Maybe I will really sell clothes and those things, or maybe set up a business to sell handicrafts, stuffed toys - a kind of store.

I haven't decided yet. Sometimes I think I will never totally retire, because if I am not going to work in the brothel anymore, I will always have my friends, my regulars, outside, they will call me on my cell phone. The new trend now is the cell phone.

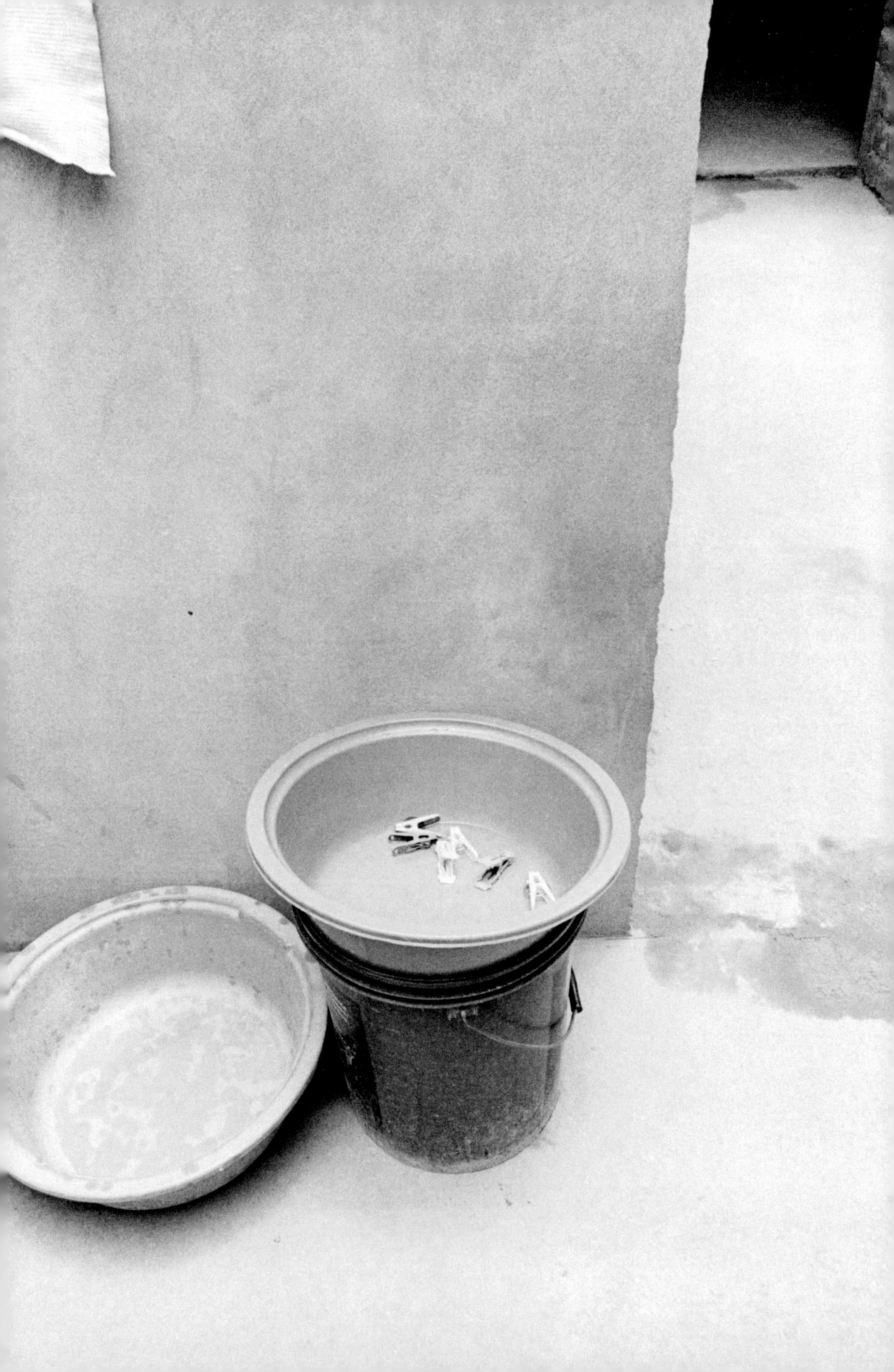

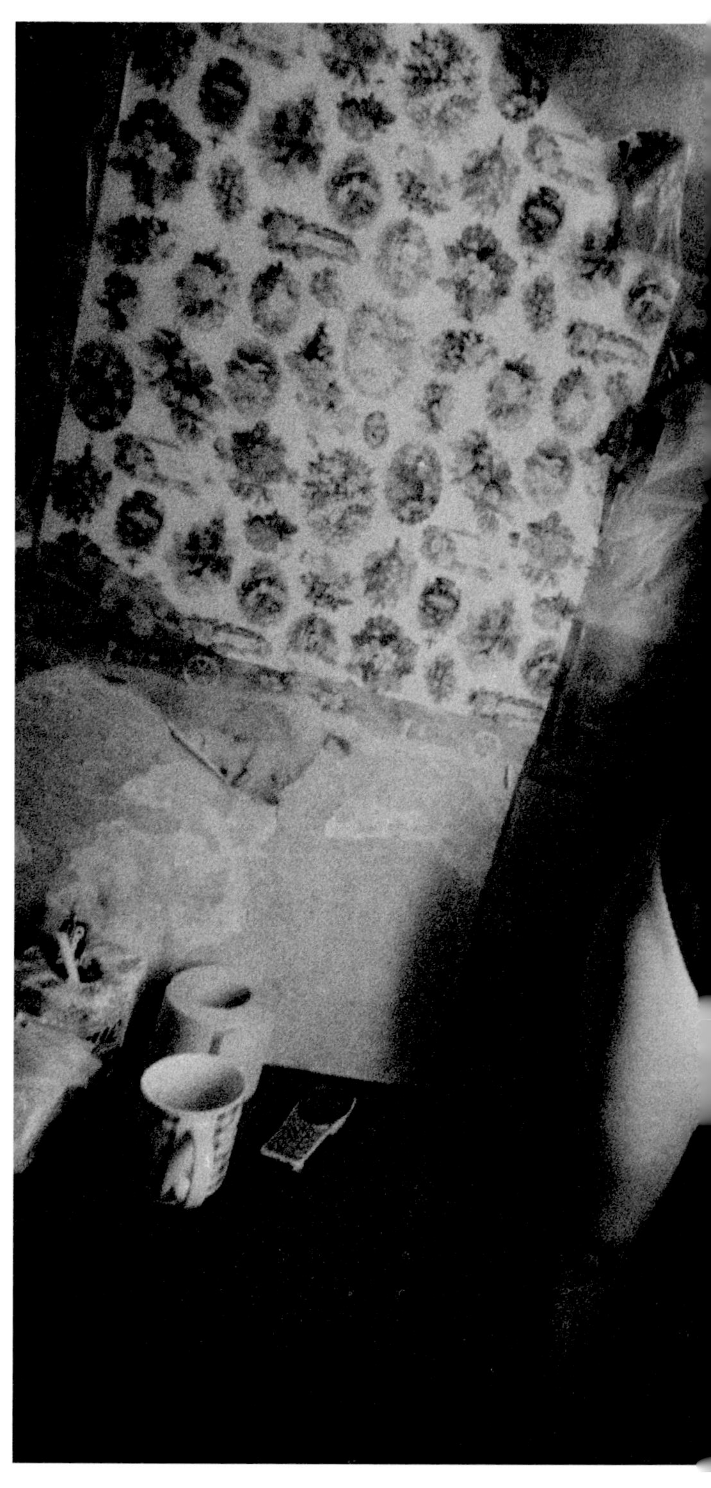

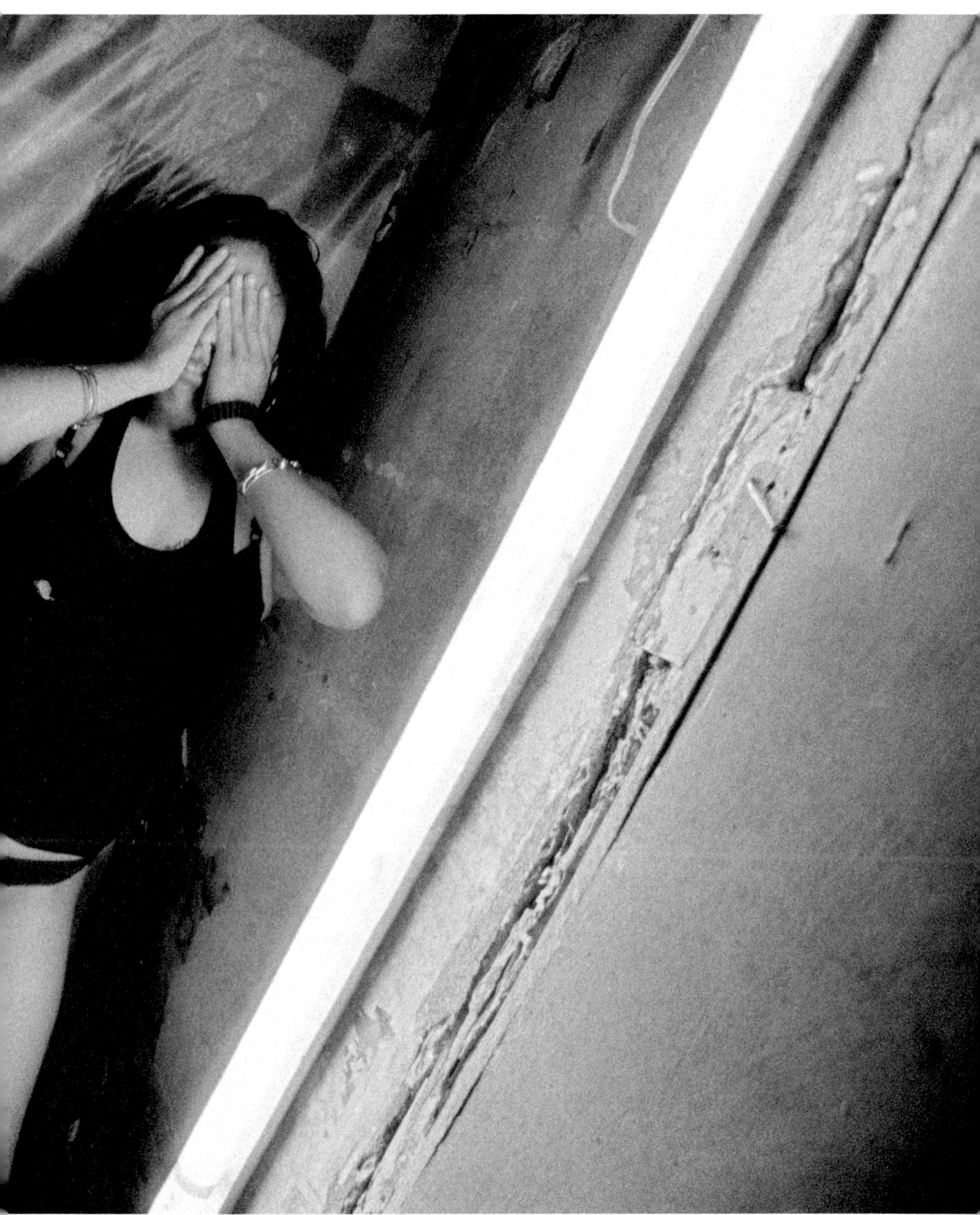

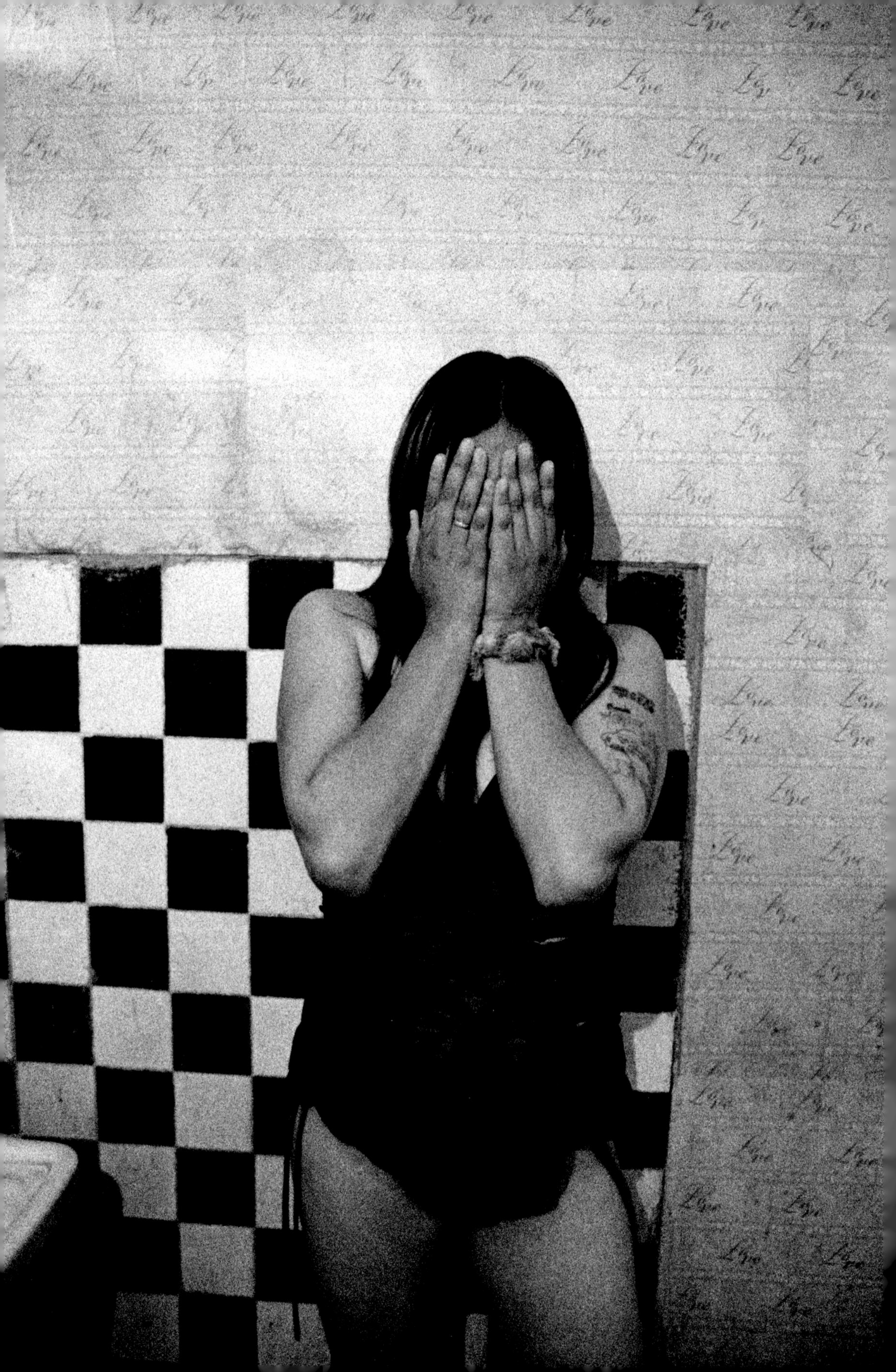

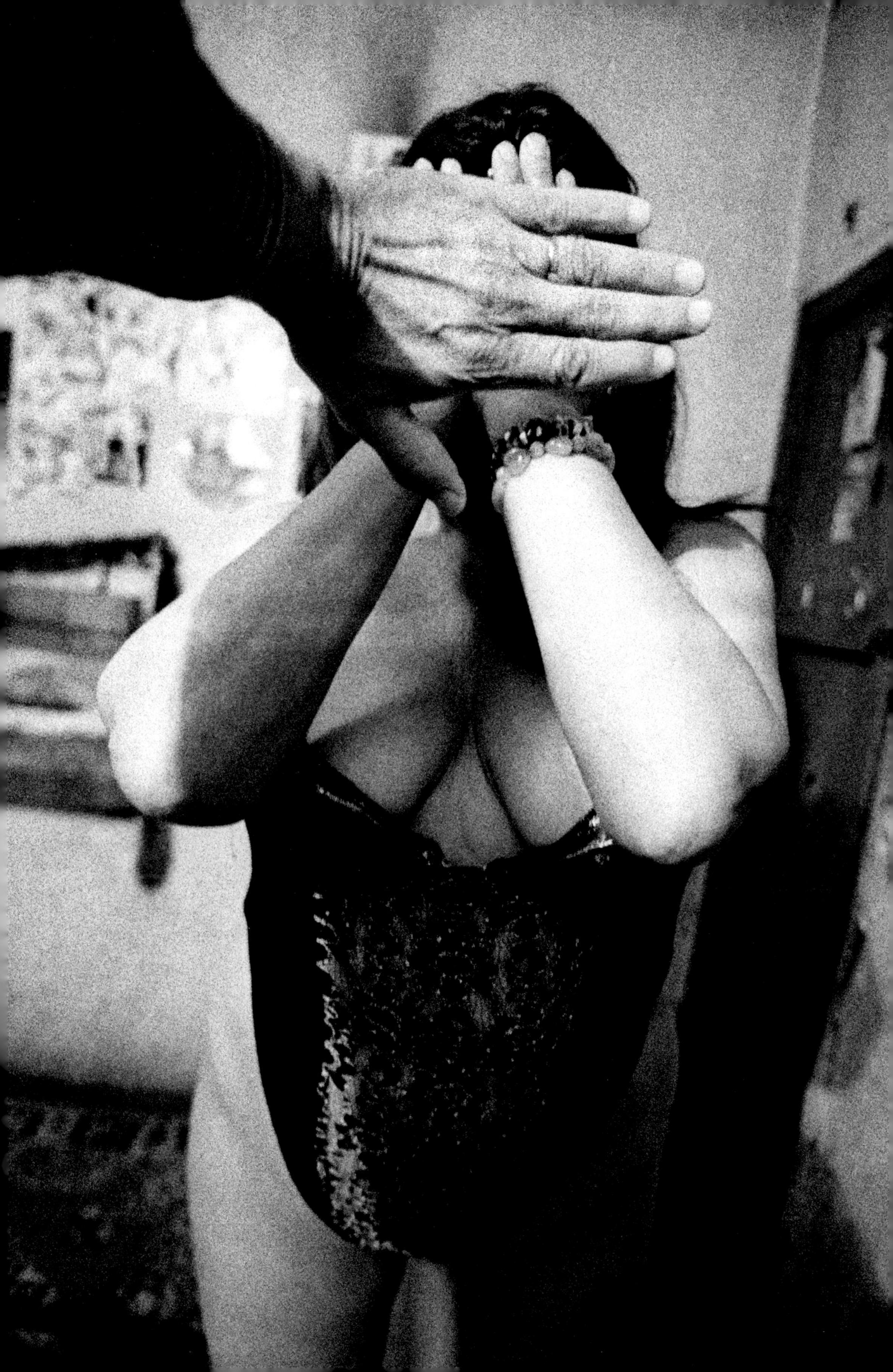

PATRICIA

49 YEARS OLD · HOUSEWIFE AND SEX WORKER
HAS 2 ADULT CHILDREN · LIVES IN CALLAO WITH THEM, HER GRANDCHILDREN
AND HER MOTHER

I became a sex worker when I was 18. I used to study and I had my goals: "I am going to be a lawyer." But we were very poor, my father died, I quit studying and became pregnant, I was a single mother. So then what was left - hunger, need - forced me into this... I started in bars, discos.

When I started, I didn't have any friends or anyone to teach me. When the first customer came in... I didn't even know how to wash him. As no one helps you, the customers themselves teach you, it is unbelievable. They teach you how to wash them and even sex poses. At that time we didn't even use condoms, there weren't so many diseases as now, like HIV... Fortunately, I never had any problems with diseases. Now we use condoms for everything and we have checkups every 28 days.

But don't think this is easy, we have to withstand shame, humiliation and abuse, from everyone: the police, and customers too... "I am paying you, that's why you have to obey me," they tell us and we have to put up with it. Some are a little bit crazy and we have to follow their games. We are even counselors because they come with their problems. In general, men mostly come to us because we satisfy their fantasies.

Two terrible things happened to me at the brothel: once when I was a young girl, a man raped me from behind, and I didn't say anything because I was ashamed. Each time I remember I feel (tearful). I wish this feeling would go away; I am sure if this happened now, I would scream and hit him.

The other one was when my brother saw me. "Shit, what do I do now?" And I hid. He disappeared. Then, back home, he didn't even ask me or reproach me; I guess maybe it was because I helped him with his studies and food. What was he going to say? Maybe it was also because I was never shameful, it was always from my house to work and from work to my house.

In this kind of work, we are like clowns, we laugh a lot, but we don't show our true feelings. It is like any other job, I don't feel unworthy because of it... I tell you I have given my family a good start in life. Why should I be ashamed? My two sons are married, I paid for their studies, I built a 3-storey house, my son lives on the second floor and my daughter on the third. My grandchildren are a beauty.

The work issue is never discussed in my family, even though I suppose my kids sense something, and because of my grandchildren, too. Each time sex workers are in the news, being taken to jail, all covered up, my daughter says, "They deserve it because they're lazy. Why don't they work?" But one day I made them watch a TV programme about a sex worker leader and her family life; since then, my children changed, they don't talk badly but they don't ask anything either. In a Lima way, I leave them clues, Urpi (Guidance and counseling center for sex workers) or Miluzka (Sex Workers Association, created for the defense of their human and civil rights with their active participation) leaflets, I speak to them about the workshops I go to, I show them pictures... I think they know. The truth is, I don't think they will reject me if I tell them, the thing is how do I tell them! In regards to Urpi or Miluzka, they are organizations that have helped us see and claim our rights, and to organize ourselves. For example, the police do not come here as they used to: One day they arrived at 3 in the morning, they wanted to shut down the place because of problems with the license. They put us all against the wall, and started shooting with their submachine guns, they treated us like criminals, as if it were a raid in prison. In addition, TV reporters came with their cameras... If we organized ourselves, we could learn to love ourselves more and face this type of despicable act, by coming forward.

Can you imagine? Coming forward? In this way I could be more open with my children, because my partner already knows. Yes, I met him at work, he was a customer! There I found this short, ugly man, but he is so nice! The girls used to tell me "Don't fall in love

here" but you see. The first years I knew him
I suffered a little because he continued with his
single life, but at least he wore a condom, ha!
ha! Until we got used to each other and now
we've been together for about 15 years. He is
14 years younger than me.

I'm already retiring from this work, I only
do it on weekends, because even though you
are productive, you wear yourself out. I get
home a little nervous. Luckily, my partner earns
some money and I have my savings with which
I can make knitted things or clothes, I would
like to help other girls with workshops so they
can learn to do the same and set up their own
company. Of course I would also like to help
them get organized to defend our rights. We
are now thinking of a way to organize ourselves.
We're still only a few but we are going to start.
In this way, every time people insult us and call
us whores, with disgust on their faces, or want
to throw us in jail, we will stop them and make
them respect us.

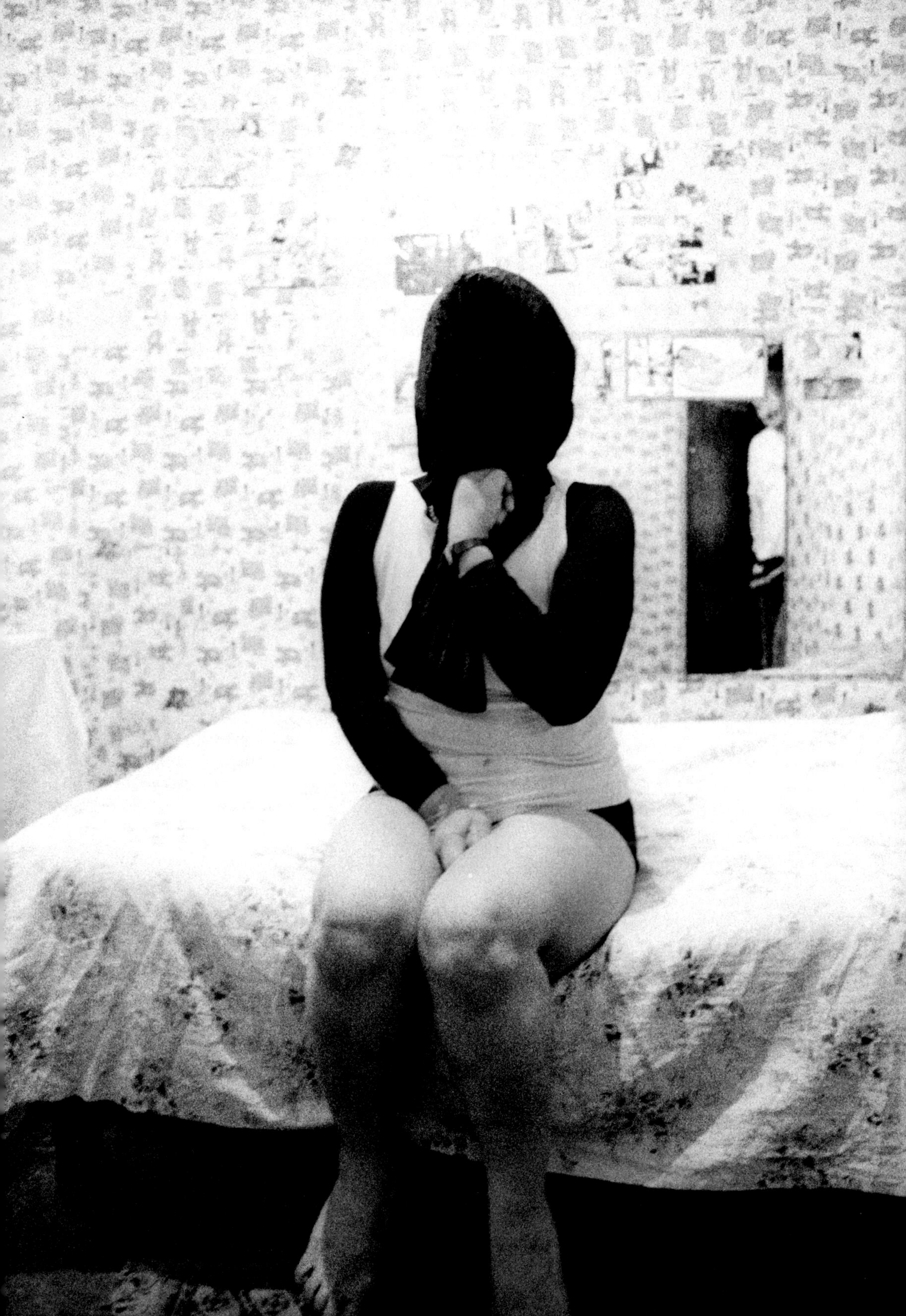

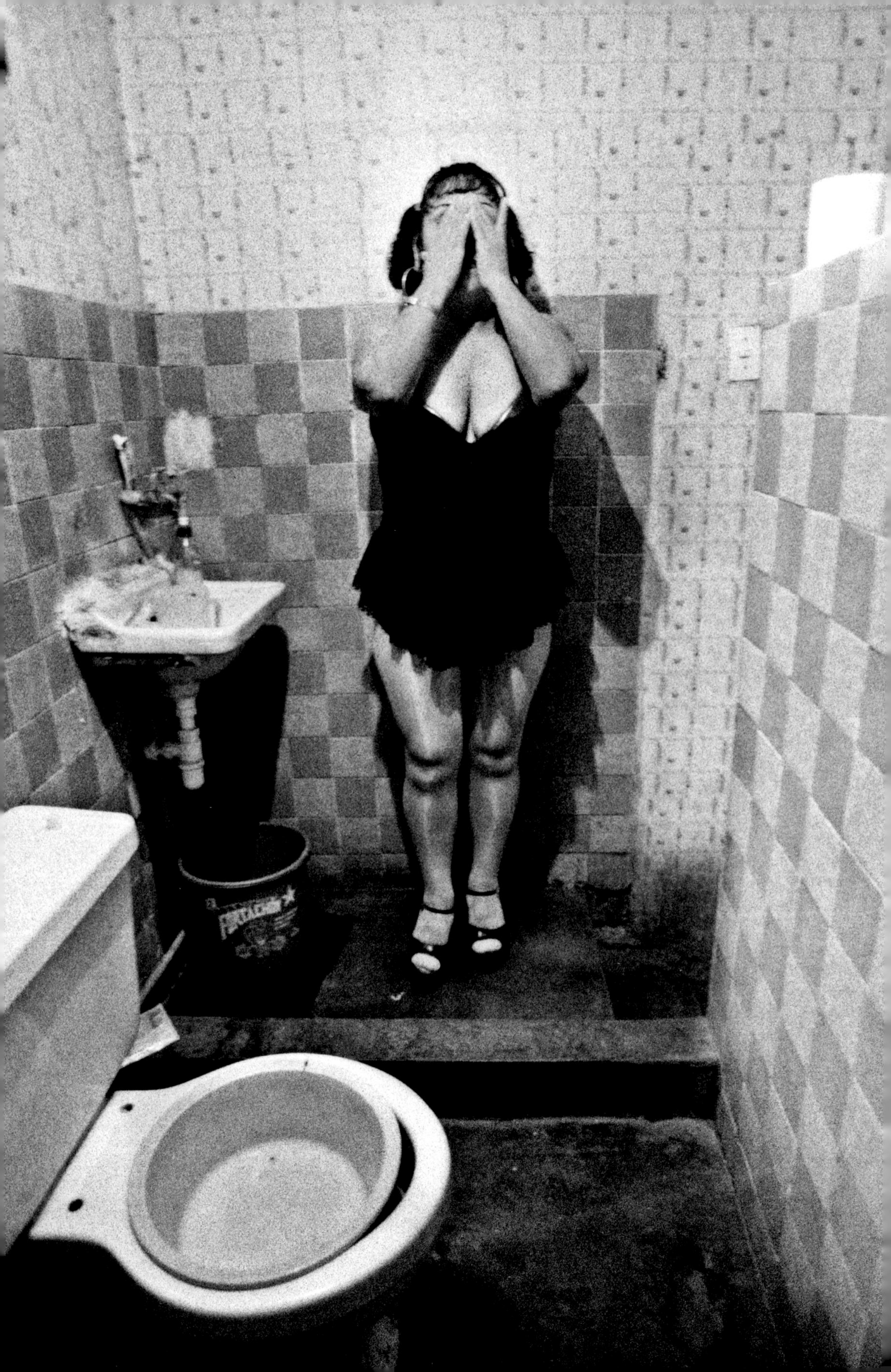

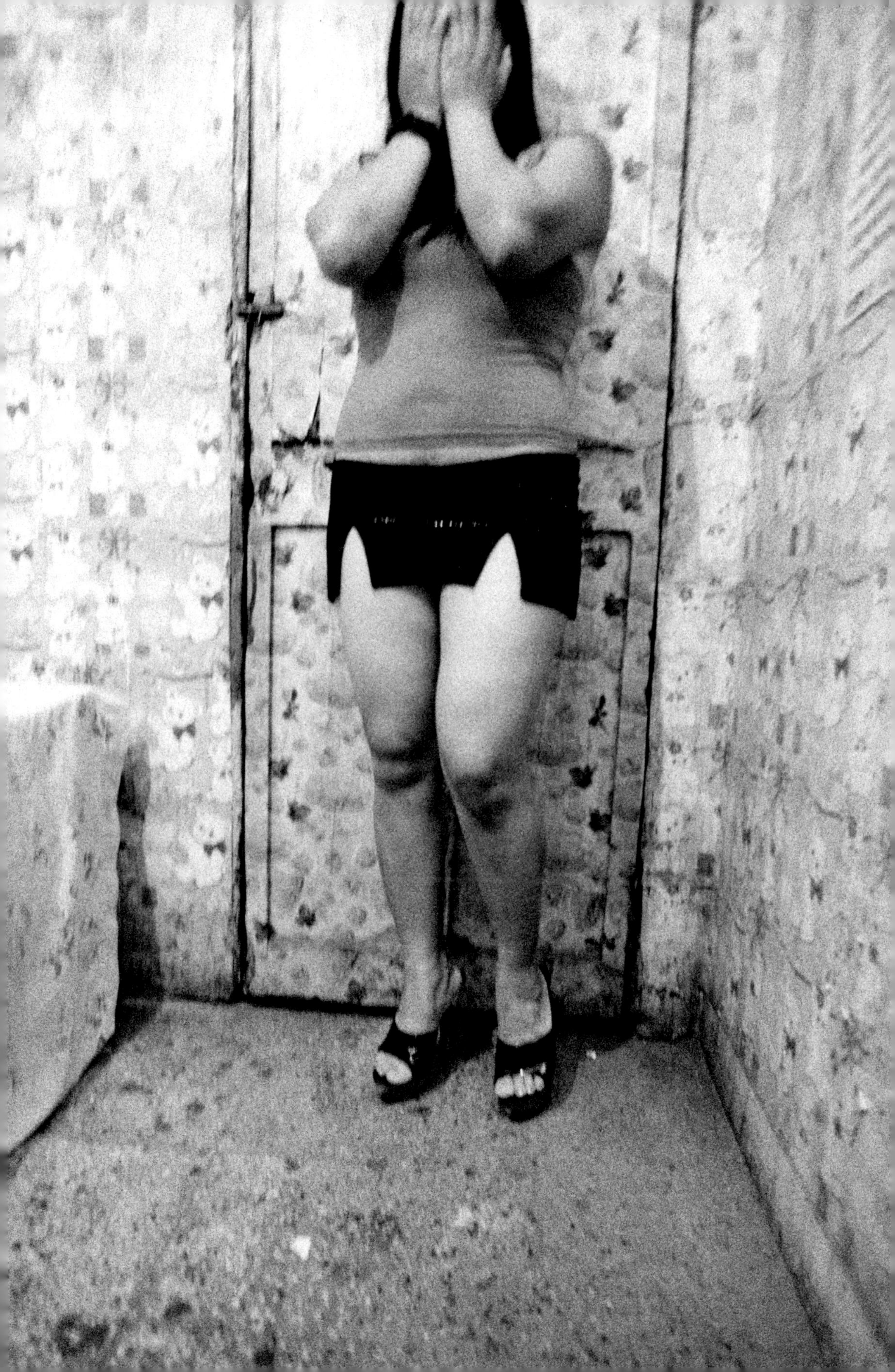

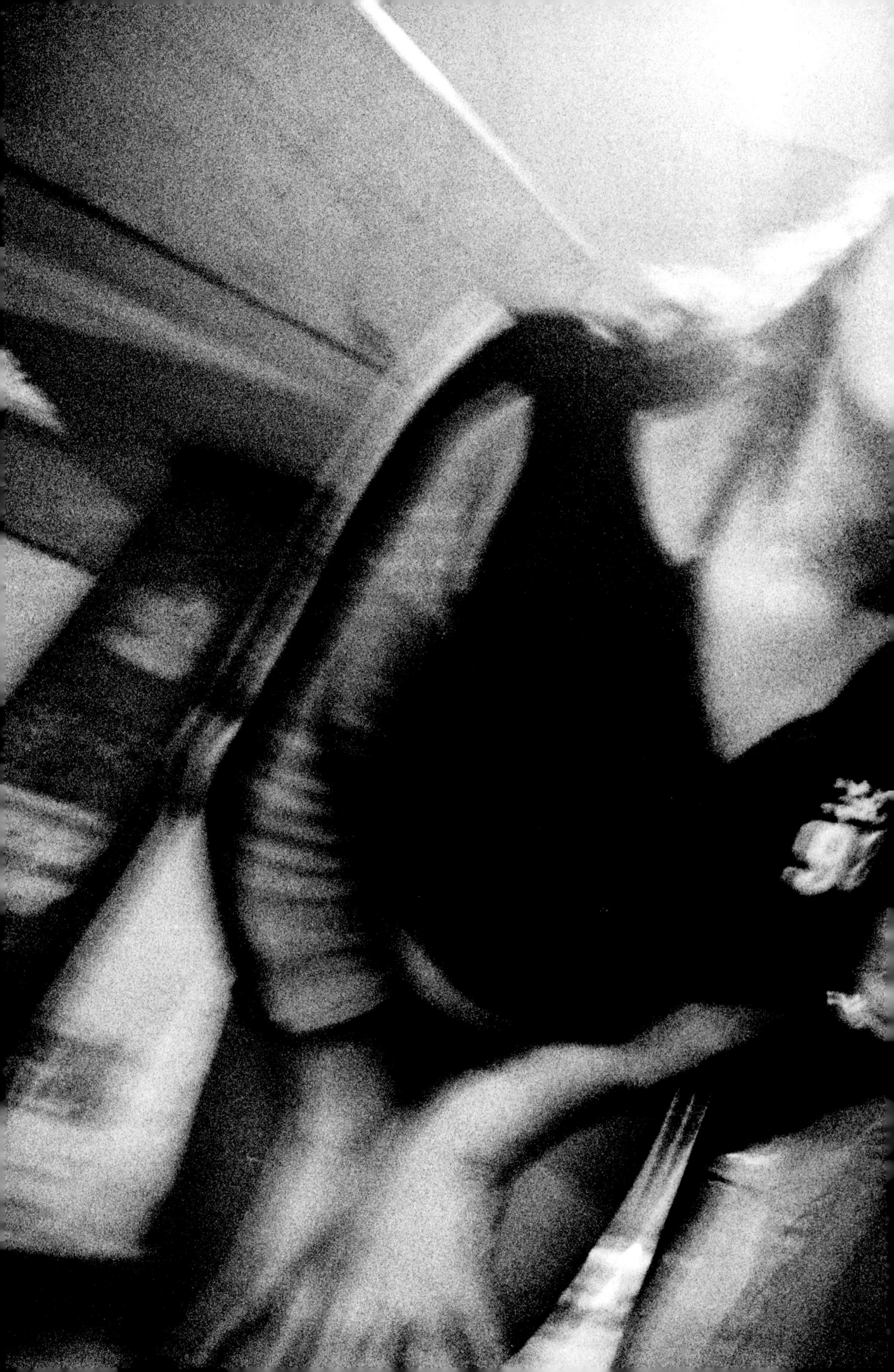

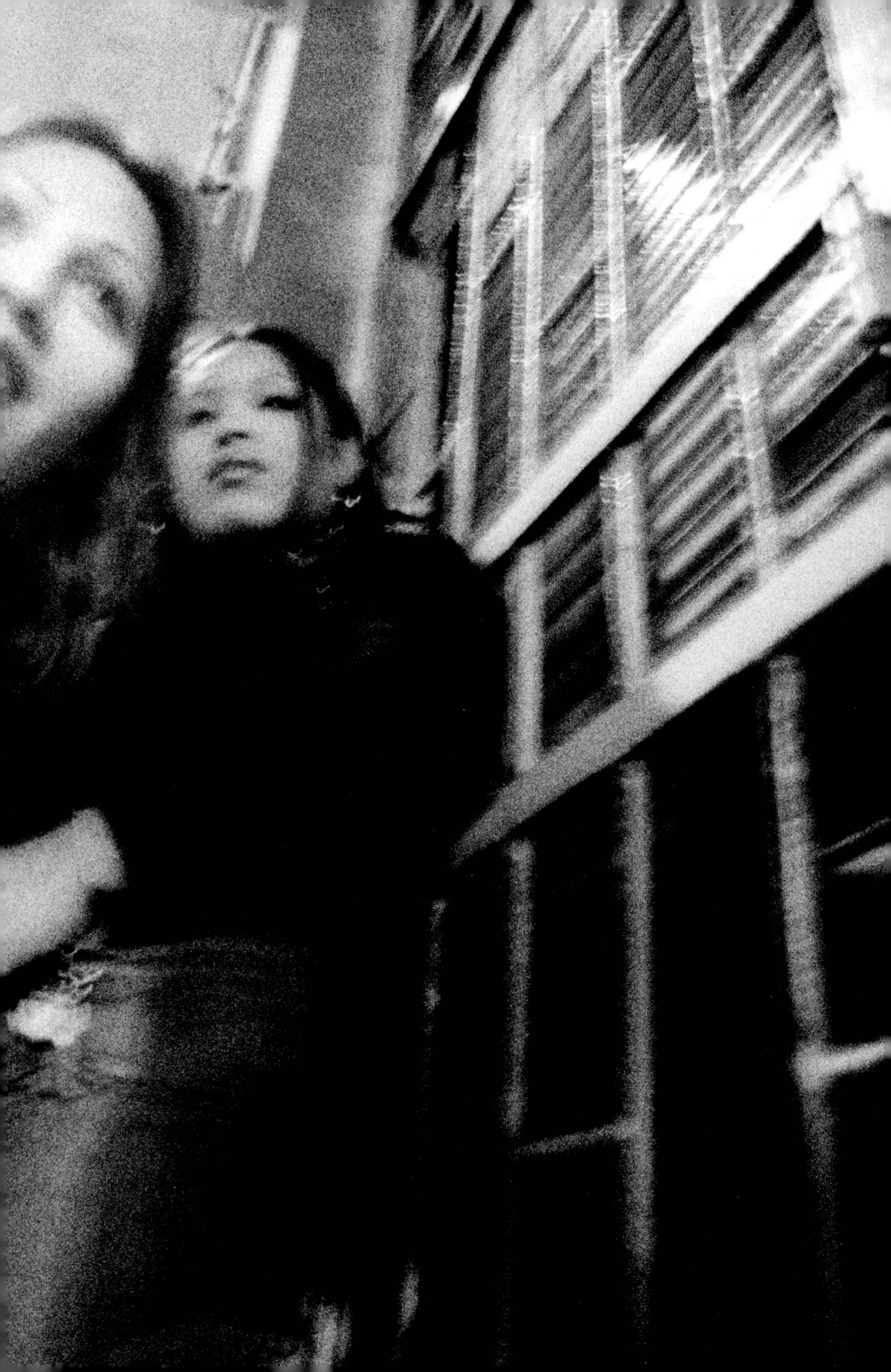

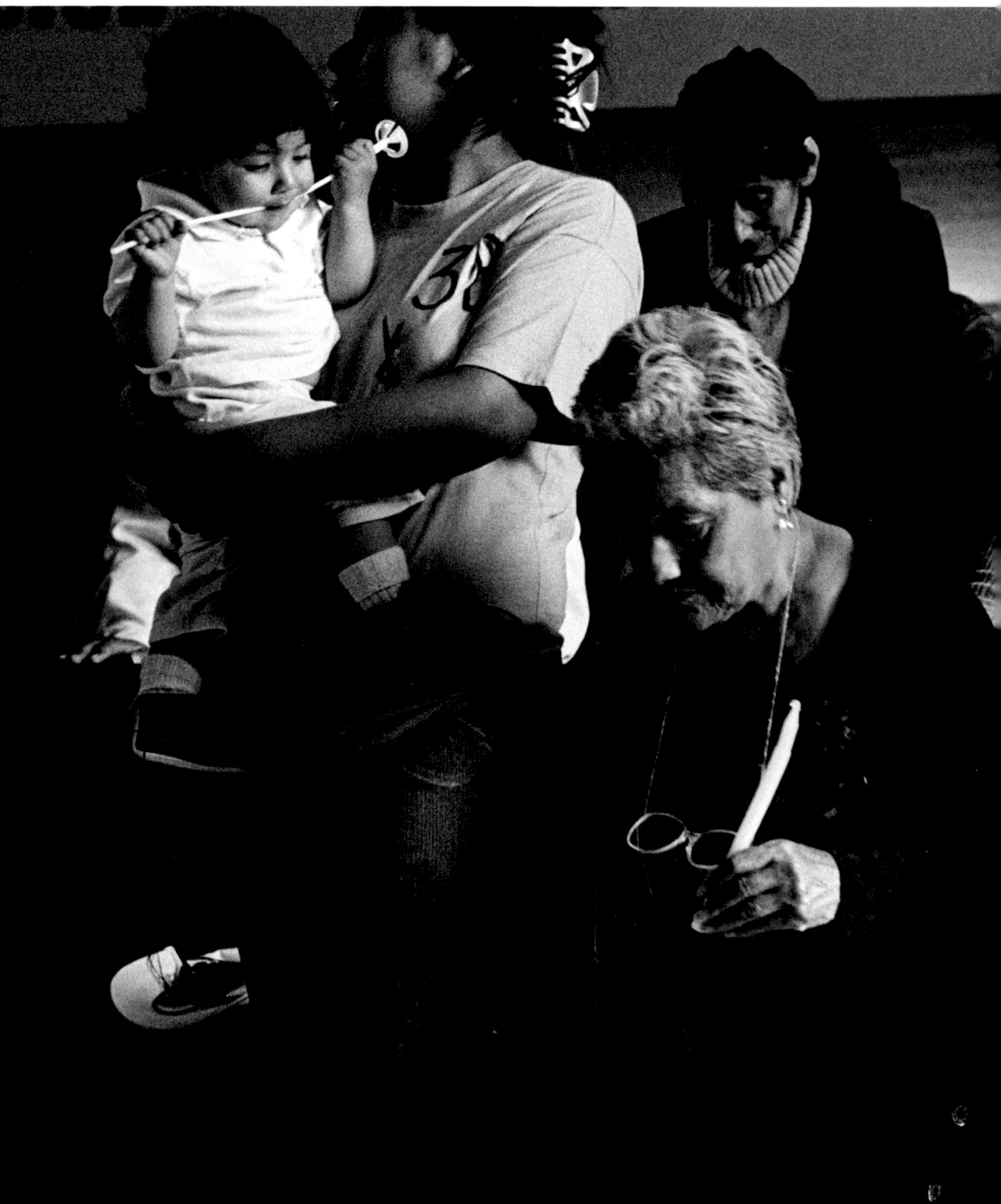

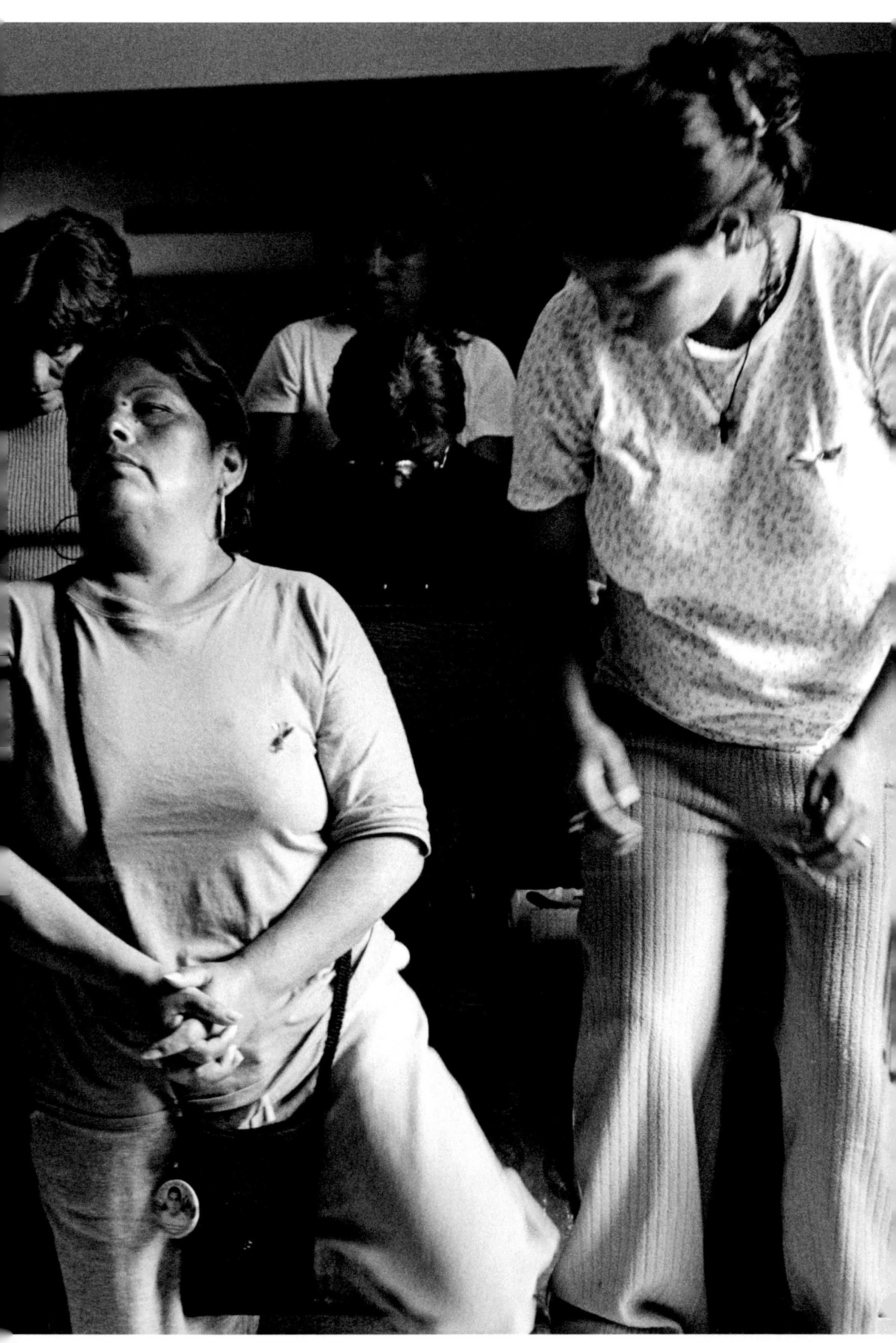

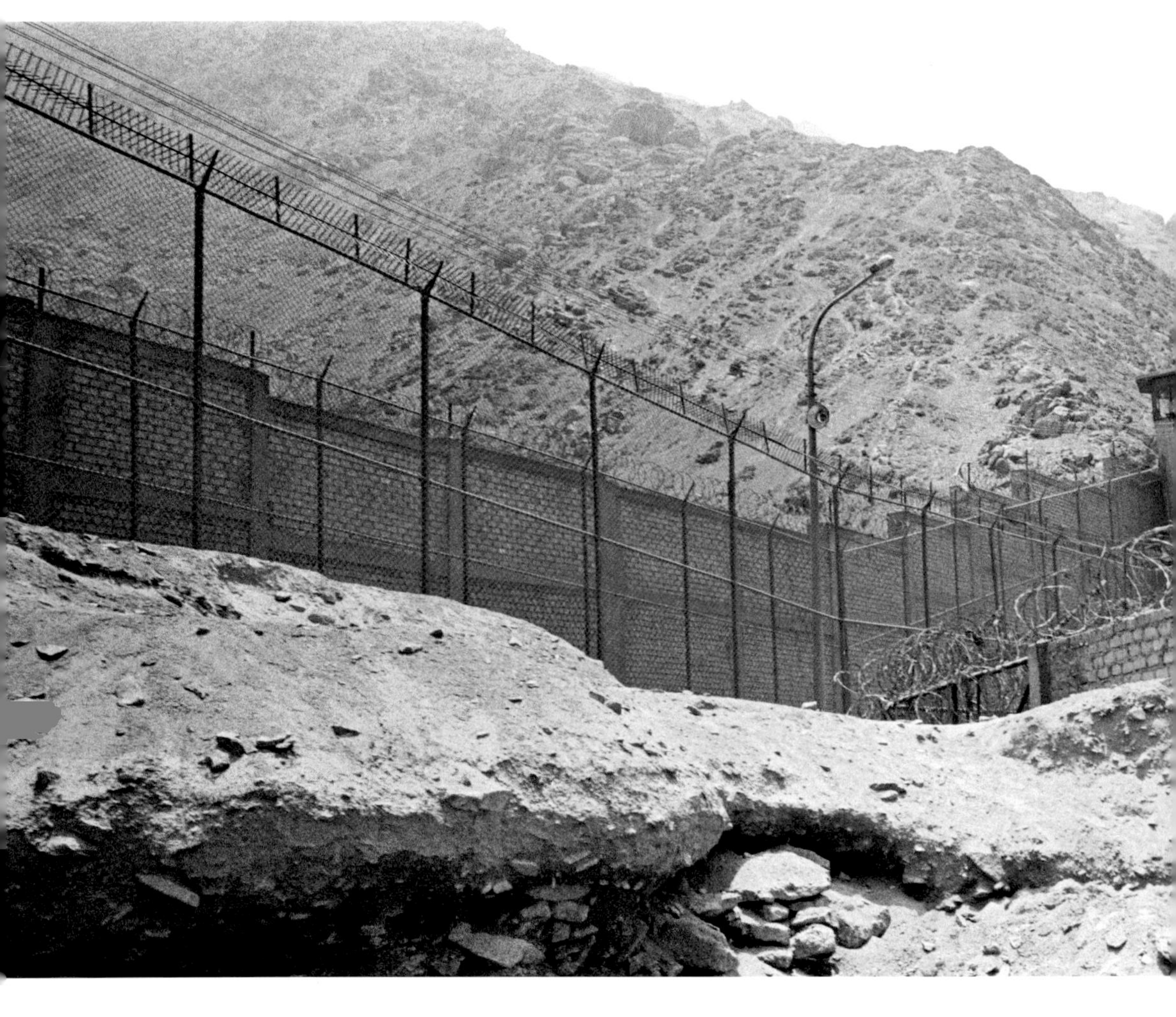

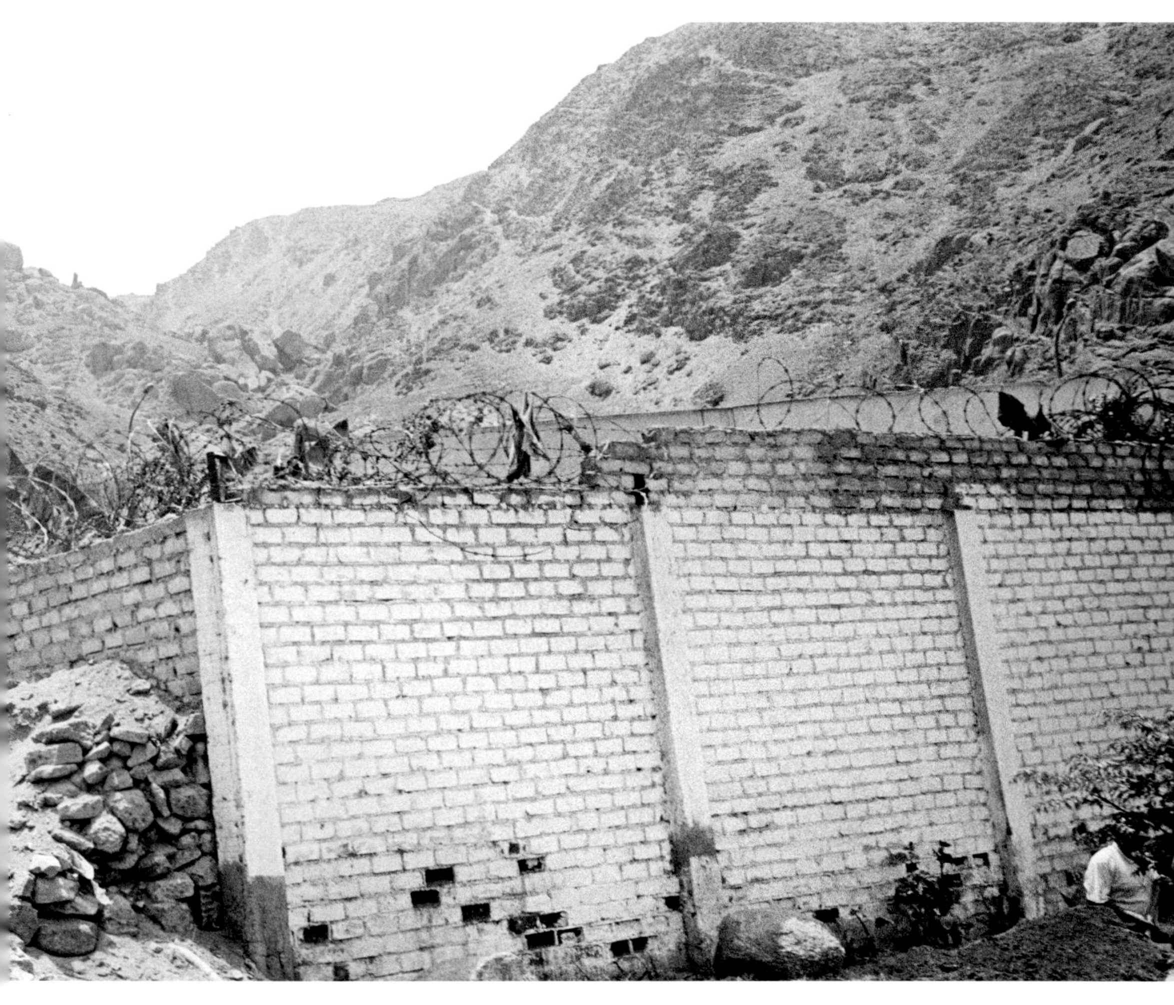

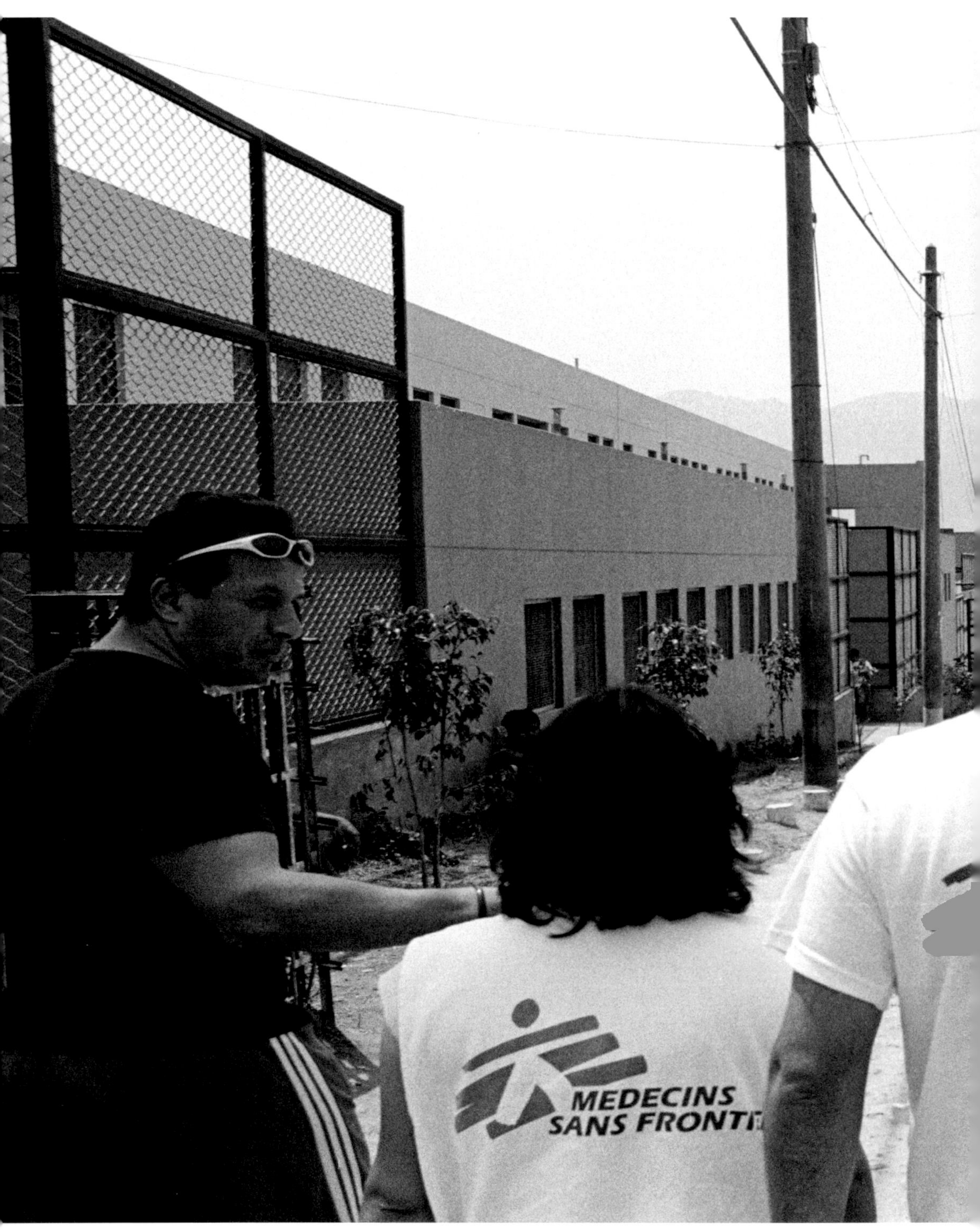

MEDECINS
SANS FRONTI

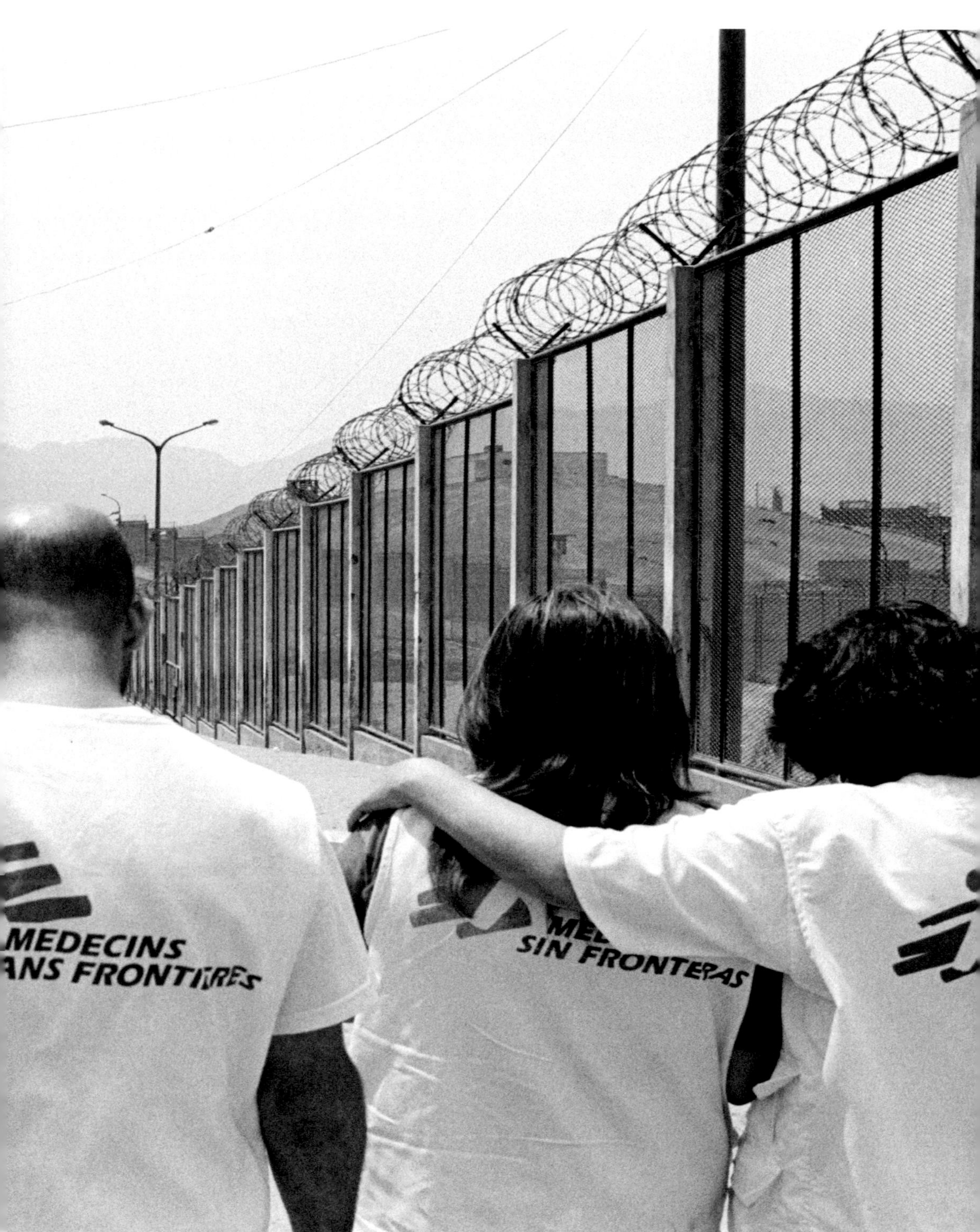

MEDECINS
ANS FRONTIÈRES
MÉDECINS
SIN FRONTERAS

Carmela

I entered Hermelinda Carrera (well known youth reformatory for girls under 18) before I was fifteen years old. My friends and I were even going to celebrate my Quinceañero (party to celebrate a girl's 15th birthday, a symbol of passing from a child to a woman). Everything was left behind, my dress, everything, but me, I lost my freedom.

I'm the second of 14 children. I never had my mother or father's love. My father was too rude and violent - he beat us with a wire or a whip, he gave us electric shocks and he kicked us with his steel-tipped boots. My mother was too weak; she didn't really care about us being abused as long as he didn't touch her. He was like that when he was sober… That's why I prayed so hard for him to become an alcoholic: when he was drunk he apologized, danced, played, pampered us and even kissed us.

When I was thirteen, I couldn't stand it anymore so I ran away. I lost my way; I slept in empty houses under construction. I covered myself with cement bags and ate leftovers. I found a job as a maid in a house. I was working there for a year when one time the owner's grandson tried to rape me. Thank God my father had taught me to fight so I could defend myself. But when I told the owner that I was quitting and I asked her to pay me, she answered, "What I am going to do is call the police." So I decided to stay and win her trust and act as if nothing had happened. One day I took all her jewelry and I ran away.

I went to live in La Victoria (over-populated district of Lima, historically known for its high crime rate), I rented a room and lived there for a while with the money I took from selling the jewelry. I began to live big, a real show-off, I bought lots of clothes, and I spent the money on junk. Then I ran out of money, so I got a job as a welder. I made-believe I was a man, I cut my hair into a really short army-style as I was very skinny; I put on a t-shirt, a jacket and I was hired. One day, I was taking a shower and the wall made of wooden boards fell down and everybody screamed: "She's a girl, she's a girl!" I wanted to disappear. Thankfully, the owner was kind and he didn't fire me because I was very good at welding.

But once I was with the people from work somewhere, and there was a police raid. I realized that the police were looking for someone, they were showing a picture, I thought that they were looking for me, that my parents were desperate, so I introduced myself. "Here I am, I'm the one you're looking for." I thought my parents would be very happy to see me, but they came and looked at me as if I were a stray dog.

At court, the judge said: "Well, girl, you have two options, you can go back to live with your parents, or you can go to the reformatory." I chose the reformatory because I expected my parents to say, "No, daughter come home with us", but they said nothing, I noticed they were even more furious with me. When the police were taking me out, I asked mother, "How are my brothers doing?" She didn't answer. I said to my father, "Are you really going to leave me here?" and he replied, "You have chosen this by yourself," and he started to yell at me.

At the Hermelinda Carrera reformatory, a nice lady came to receive me. I was looking at my mom and crying. I wanted to throw myself on the floor and scream: "Please mommy don't leave me alone!"

That's how I got there. The day of my fifteenth birthday, I fought with a masculine girl. She was annoying me; she got on my nerves so much I got really mad. We fought in the red courtyard. She started bouncing at me so I knocked her down. Her girlfriends jumped on me. They scratched me. I crawled to a bathroom. I was so angry that I took an aluminum bucket and I went back hitting all of them with the bucket on their heads, there was blood all around, and I was in shock. The guards came, and as I stepped back, I crashed against a large window causing the glass to fall down over me. I grabbed a piece of glass and decided to cut my jugular but I didn't know where it was! I wanted to die I was so exhausted… Then the psychologists showed up, she asked me to calm down and I screamed to her, "They fuck me up for everything! They fuck me up for everything!" She sent everybody out and I felt really scared; I started hitting myself against the floor. I was so furious because of my parents, why they had left me there with people I didn't know at all. When I woke up I was in the clinic area.

That was my fifteenth birthday, it was so dreadful. I woke up, went to the bathroom, looked at myself in the mirror and promised myself that I would never, ever allow anybody to touch me again.

Since then I think to myself, "I don't love anybody." I believe that because of my childhood I'm so hard on myself, I'm like a fakir, suffering and suffering, but I can't escape from it. I would like the world to listen to my story - parents must talk with love to their children, children need to be loved, they need to have a lot of communication. There must never exist mothers and fathers like mine.

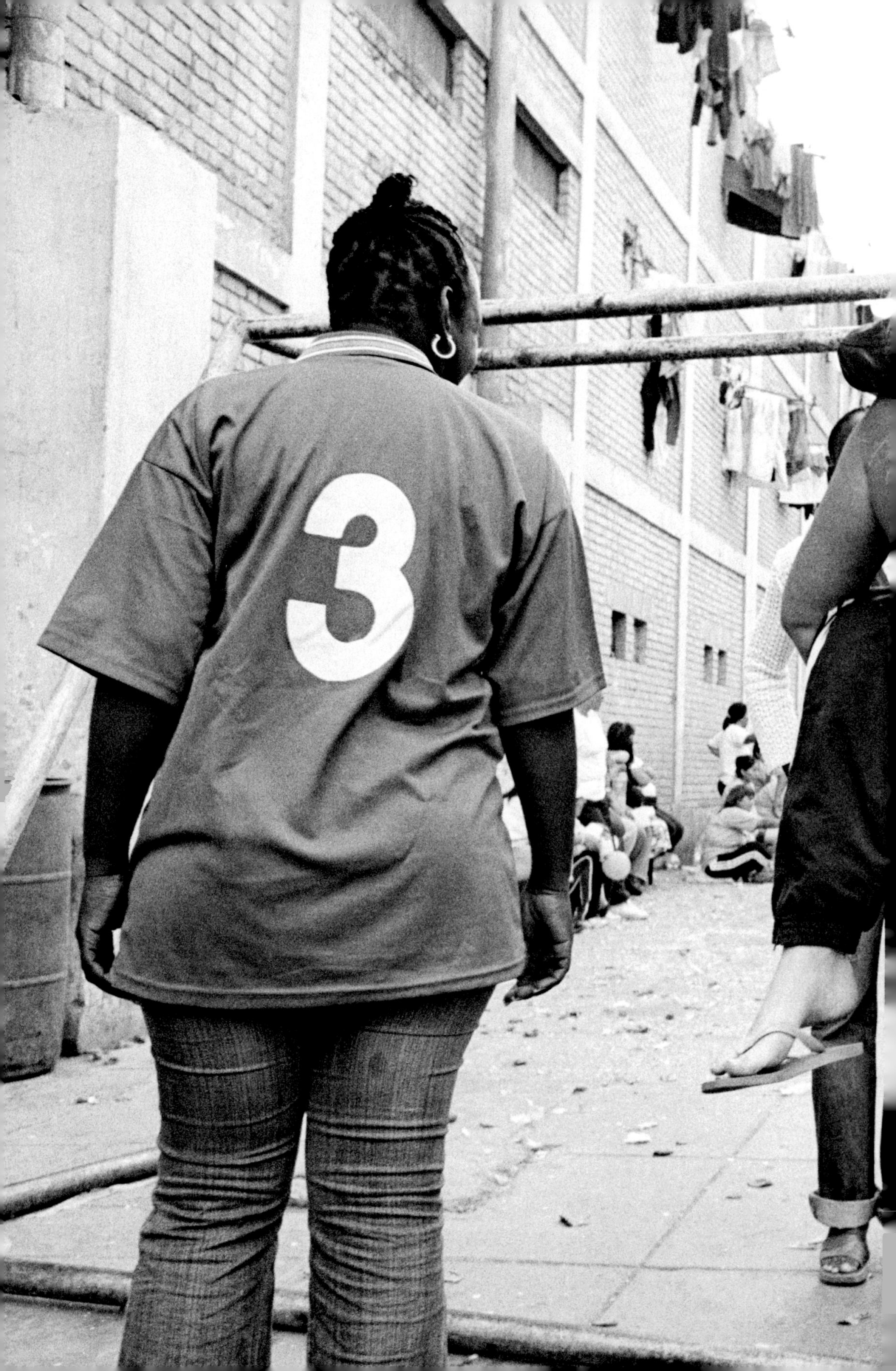

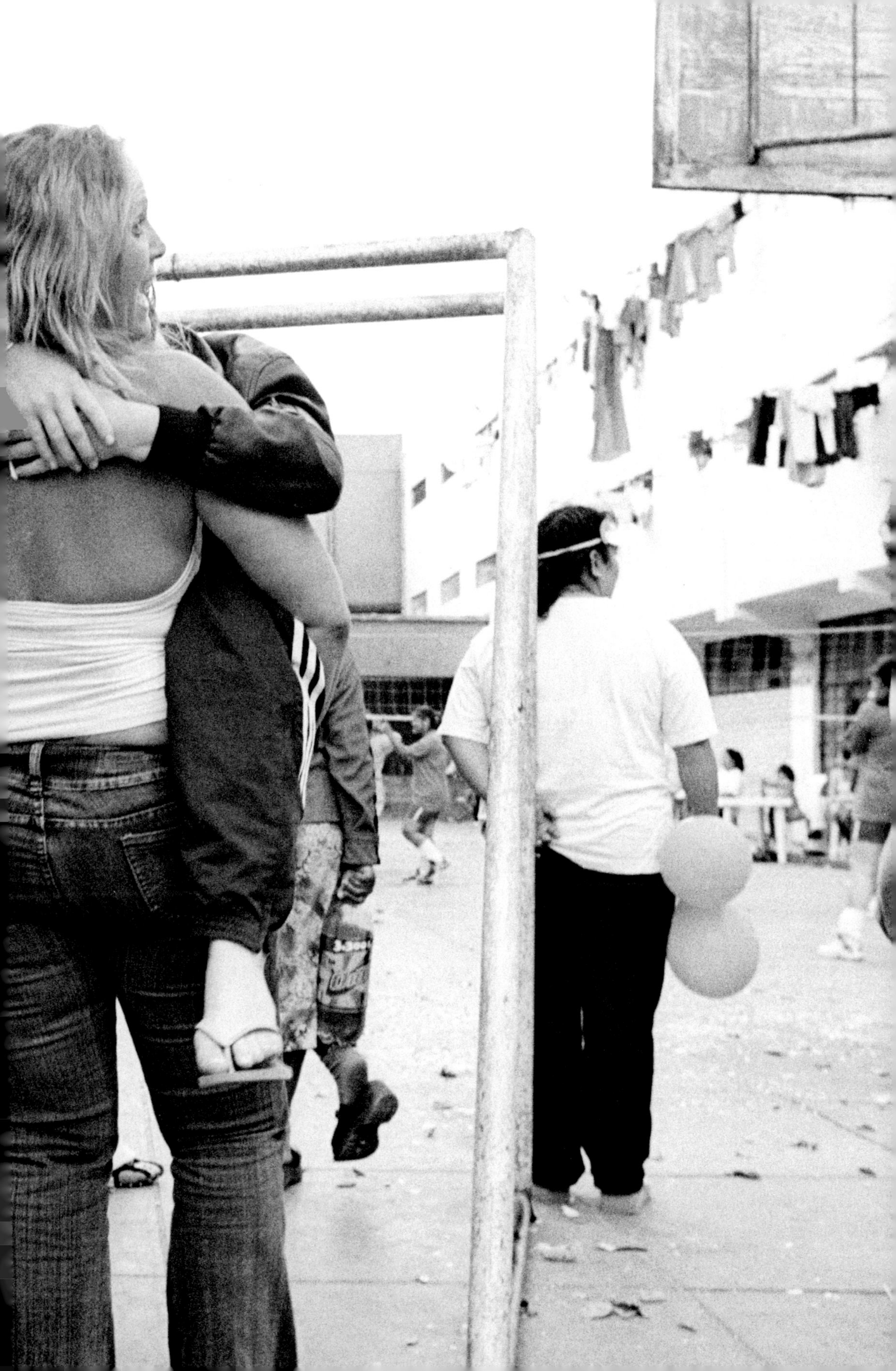

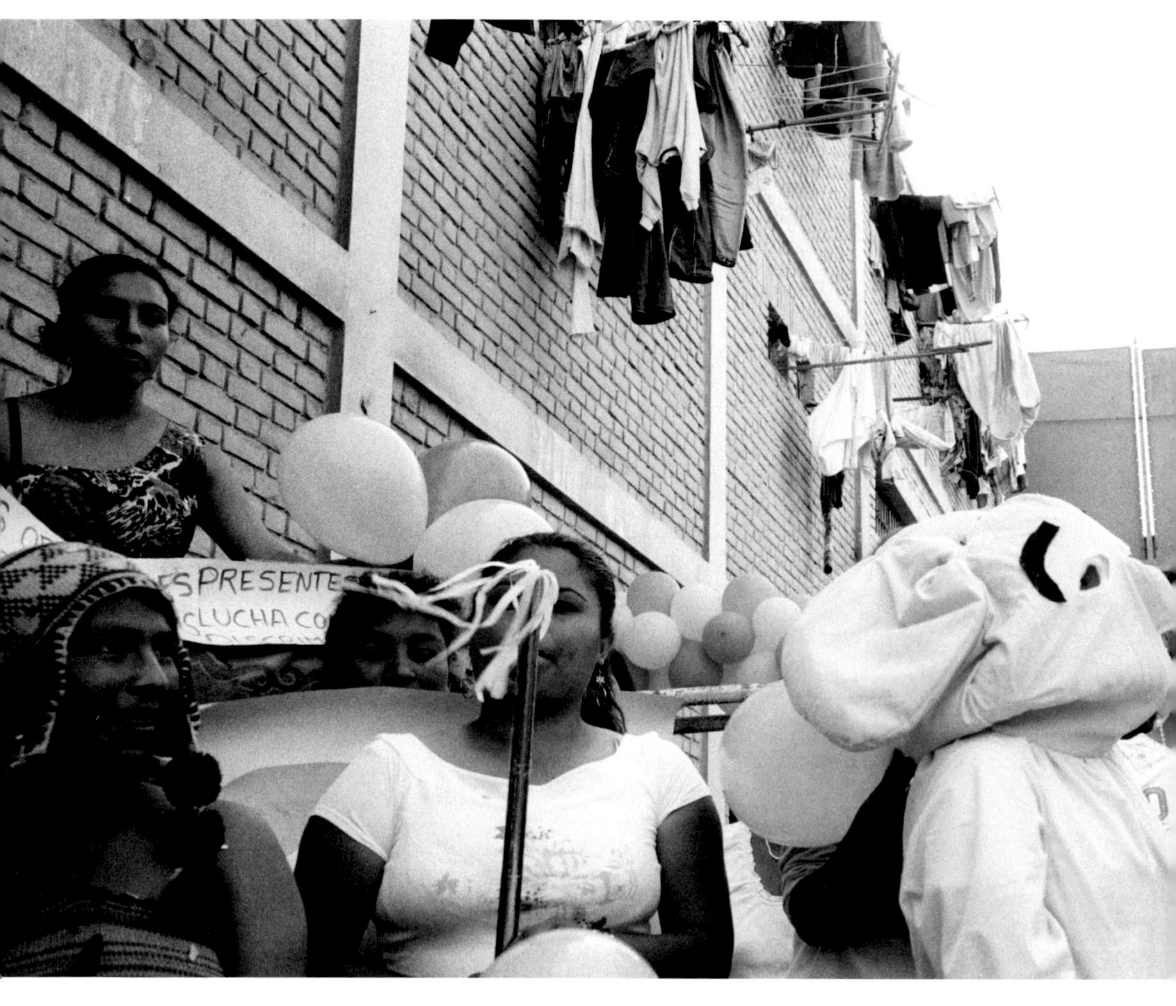
S PRESENTES
LUCHA CO

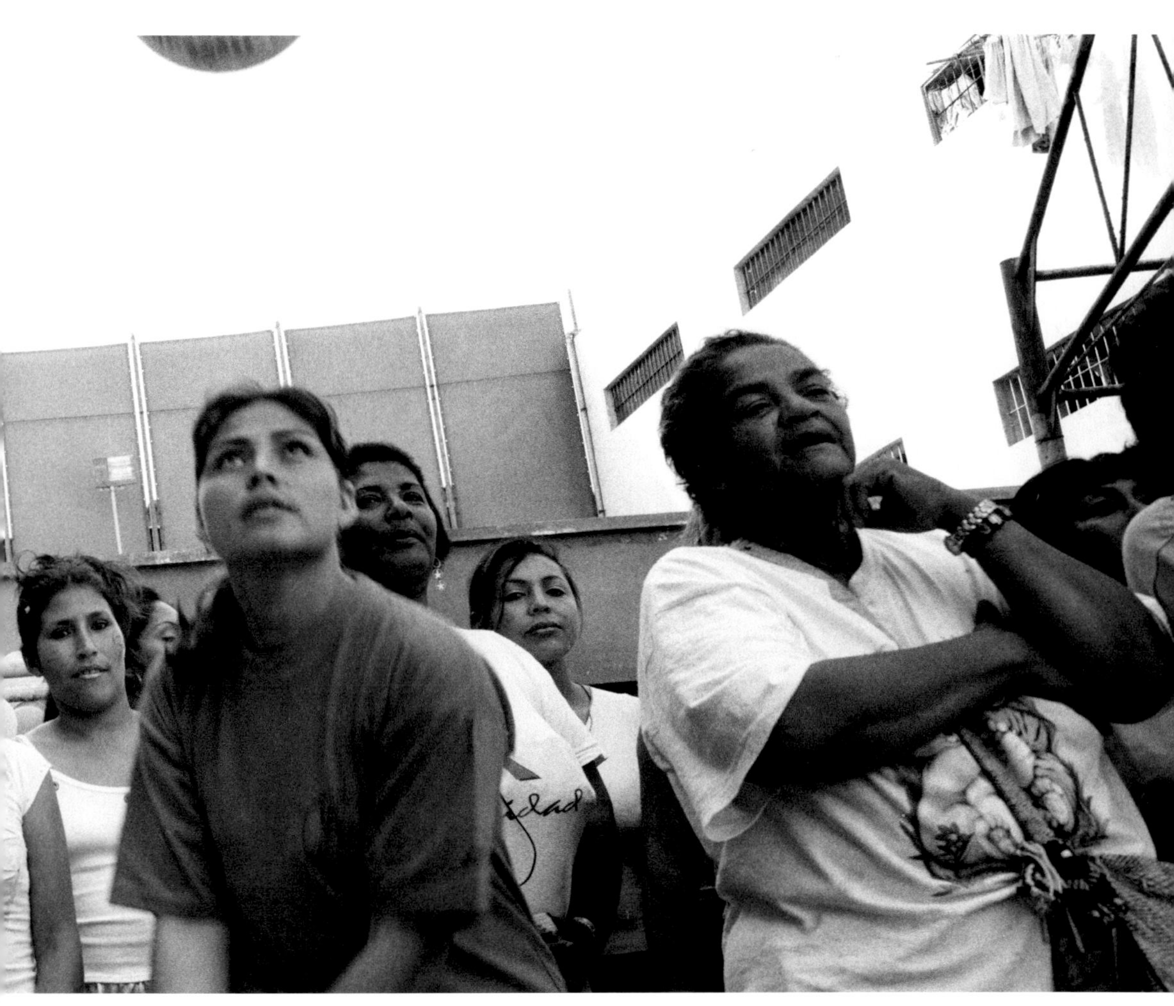

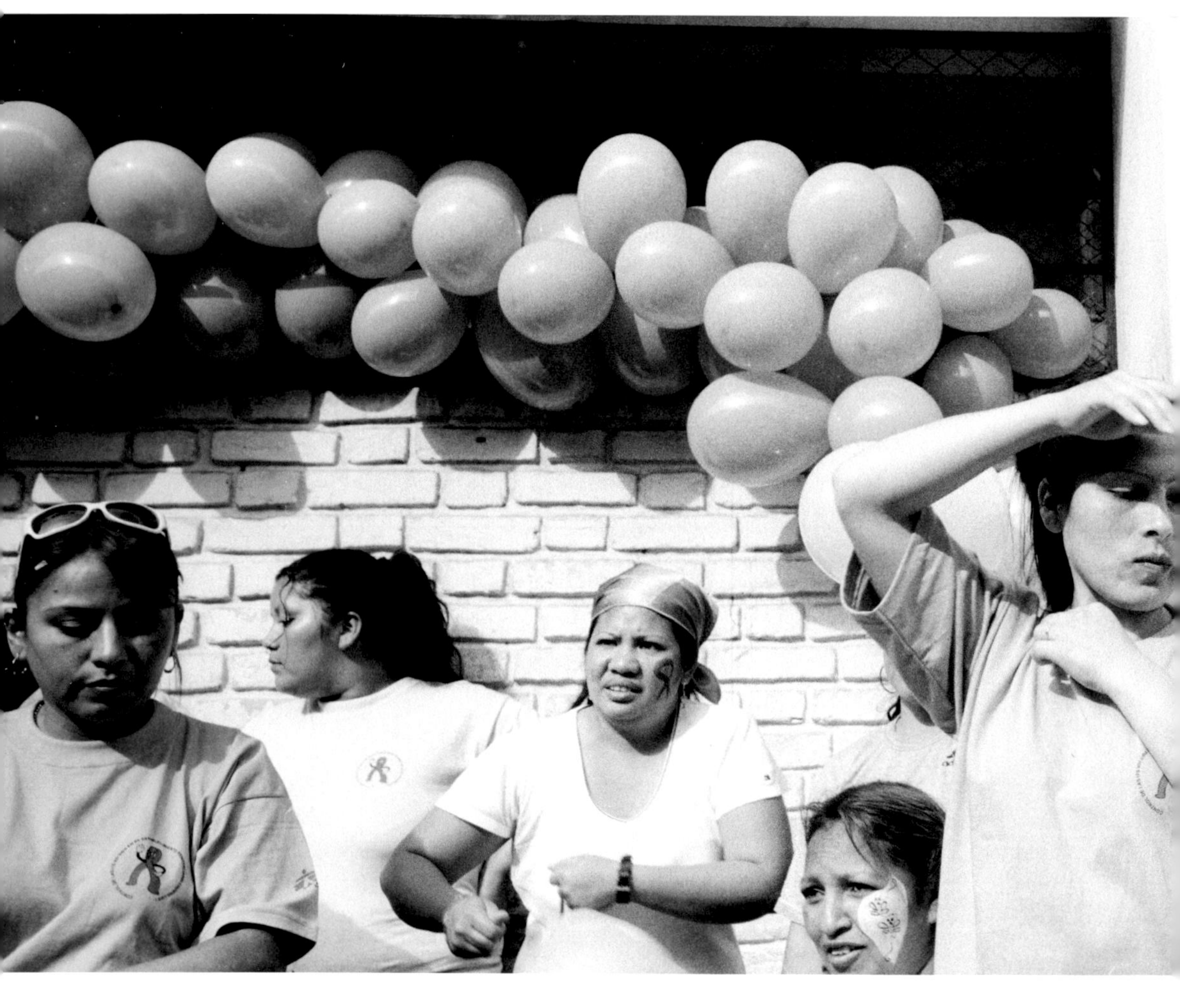

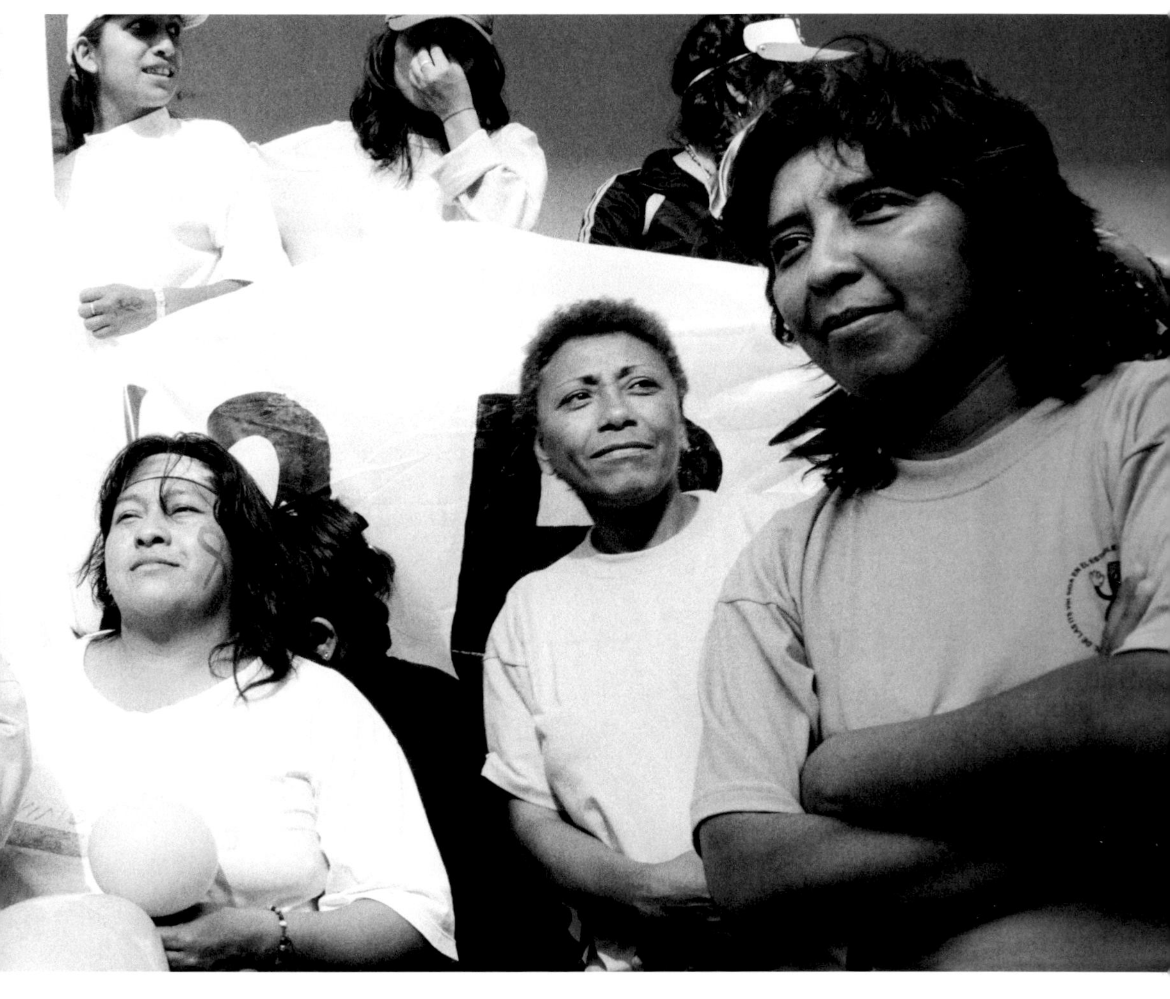

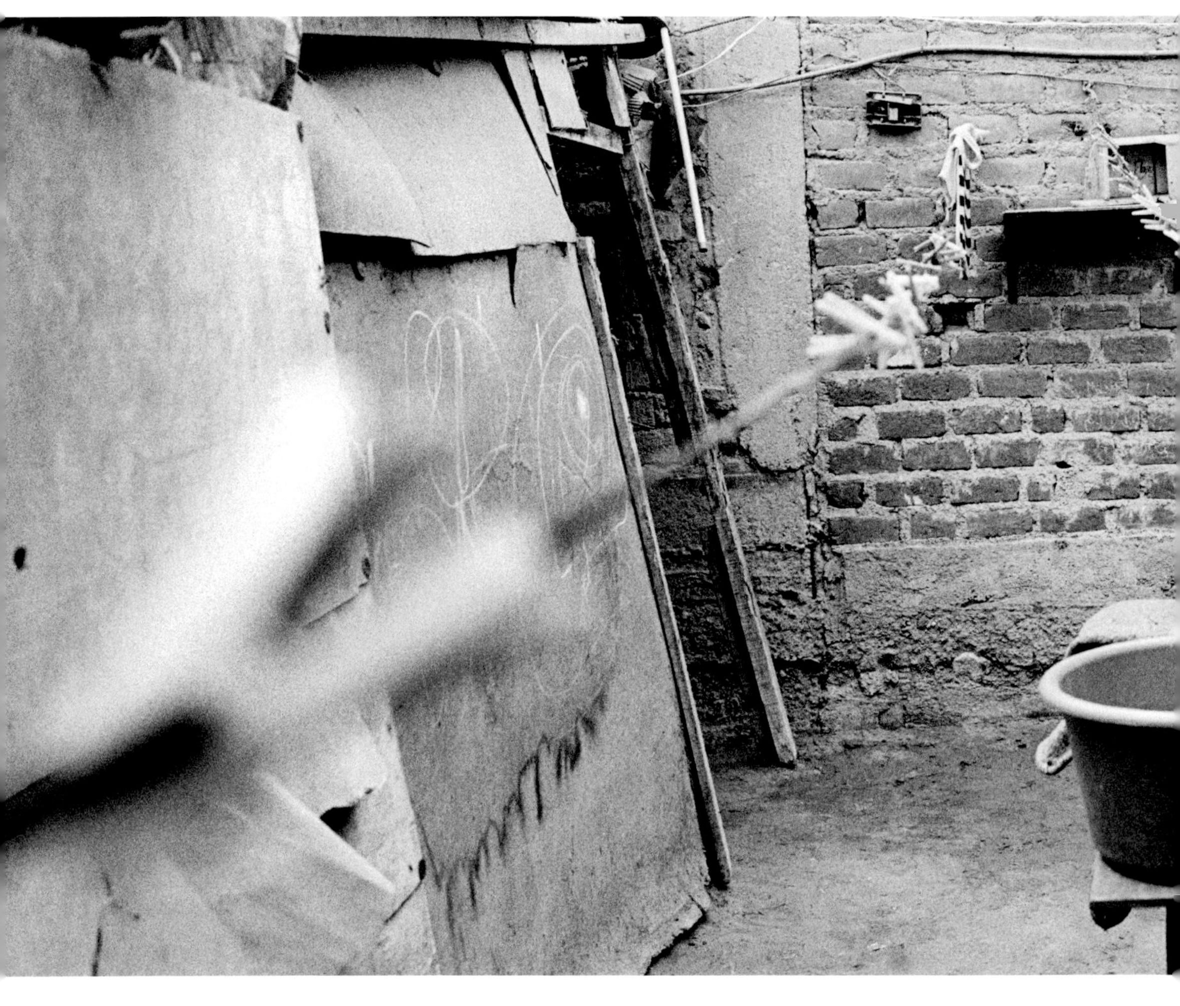

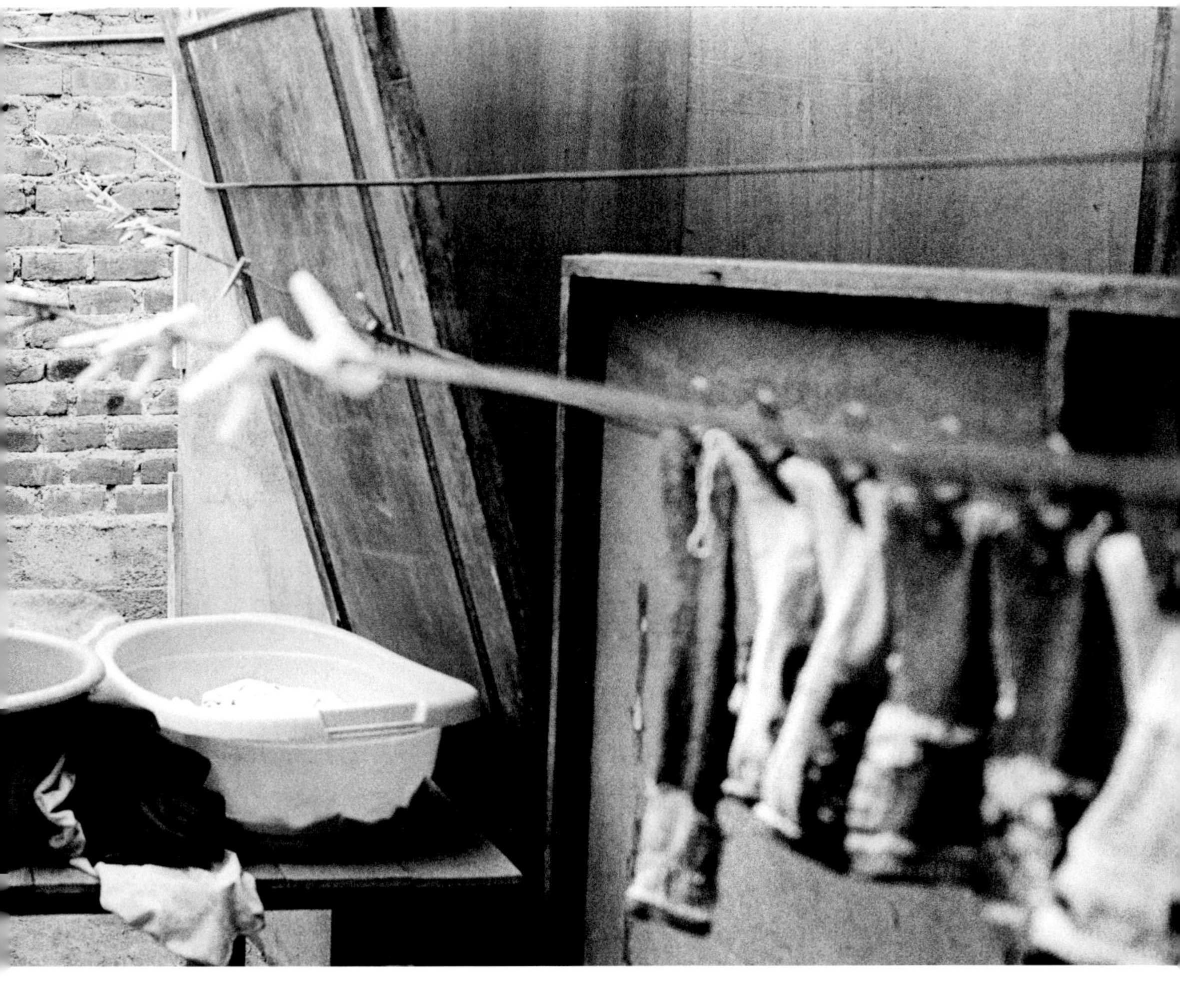

Lizeth

Sometimes I make myself believe that there is no disease in me (HIV), it's only when I fall in love I say, "Damn it! I have the disease, if I tell him about it, he may run away." Once a guy wanted so badly to be my boyfriend that I ended up saying "I am going to tell you the truth, I have AIDS". He said he didn't care. I answered, "Are you out of your mind? You have children; you should be worried about them!" He repeated he didn't care, I was so happy, I felt loved for who I was. But soon I got sick of him and I started treating him badly and liking it.

I became aware I had HIV when I was pregnant. My son's father apologized to me, "I infected you, I know you Lizeth, it's all my fault," because I wasn't dating anybody else, I was always at home. The following day, we acted as if nothing had happened. I didn't leave him, I married him. He died two years ago. I really didn't think about my disease, but my husband's. I lived for him. For example, I used to wake up at 5 am to make him breakfast, I also used to take his lunch to the bus stop. He was a Cobrador (person who receives the money in a minibus used for public transport in Peru).

But I didn't care too much about my son. My mom said to me, "You are always caring for your husband, but what about your son?" I never brought up my son well; only now because I am here locked in jail. My mother was always looking after him, I didn't have any feelings as a mother for him; I smacked him, I wanted to go out with my friends but I couldn't because he cried and I had to look after him. But after some time I realized that I must live for him because he was the only thing I had; if not, I would be alone, nobody would care about me.

When my little son was born, he was okay, but soon at five months old he started to get sick, first pneumonia, then every single disease. They told me to wait until he was two, to be sure. When he turned two, he got a positive HIV test. Before the second test (to confirm the diagnosis) I was praying, but it was positive again. It really hurt me because I thought, "I'm not important anymore but my children, sure, they are!"

Now that it is my second visit to jail, nobody comes to see me, I just talk on the phone with my family and my son. I am afraid he will get seriously ill. I call him and he says, "Mom, I am going to kindergarten, please buy me my backpack," and I feel powerless because I have no money to give him.

The first time I went to jail, my mother, my sisters and my mother's family came, but as I went back a second time, they asked me, "Why again?" I would like my mother to come and hug me and tell me how much she loves me… She just says it in the letters she sends, small pieces of paper, but never on the phone, and she never says she misses me. She says she'll come on Sunday on visiting day, I change clothes, I wait for her, but she doesn't show up…Then I think, maybe it's better because that means they are taking care of my son, but I feel so angry inside.

Once they came with my son, he said, "Mommy I love you," and I told him, "How come you love me if I smacked you because I wanted to go out, and I left you at home?" He said, "I forgive you mom"… I swear it really hurt my soul. I believe I am here in jail paying back for all I have done to my son, but I am going to change, alone as I am, I am going to get out of this, and I'll have another kind of life, I'm going to work, I am not interested if I don't make much money.

Now, my mother looks after my little son, but when she was locked up in jail, it was really hard: my sister, who is now 22, couldn't take care of him because whenever she had to take my son to the hospital she didn't know what to do with her own children… then I left my son with my aunt but she didn't really care about him, he was dirty all over and I was afraid she would forget to give him his medicines… then I took him to my mother-in-law's but she has many grandchildren and she works just next to a rubbish dump and my poor little son was always there.

Finally I sent him to my father, because his family is doing better than my mother's, but it became difficult for my father to take him to the hospital, to give him the medicines, to take care of him, but the worst thing was that he had a monkey at home. One time my father showed up at the prison, he had never come before. He told me that my son had been bitten by the monkey and I panicked thinking about my child's disease but my father asked me, "Why are you crying?"… So I had to tell him about my son's disease and I asked him to get rid of the monkey… but he said: "Now the monkey is infected." You can't imagine how much that hurt me.

Once they asked if I had AIDS, I always denied it: "No, no, no, no." I never tell the truth. People discriminate because of their ignorance. When I hear people talking like that I don't say a word, I believe that if I weren't HIV positive I would say, "Why are they talking like that?" However, as I know I am HIV positive I say nothing because I don't have the courage.

All of my family know about it, I told my mother's family so they could help me… They don't help me too much but at least with diapers for my child, so I don't have to go out to steal. From my father's family side, no one helps me.

It started when I was twenty-two… when my son's father was alive I didn't have to ask for milk for my child. He bought everything for my child. He never bought only one diaper; he used to buy diaper packages. When he died, that was it, I had no money left, my husband's family didn't help me, my mother's family, they did, but they only brought me three diapers.

I had a fifteen-year old sister and she helped me a lot because she used to steal, and she put me in touch with her gang. One day my sister didn't go with them to rob, so I called one of them and I asked him to take me instead. It started then. At first, I did nothing, I just sat in the car while they divided up the stolen money. They all got 500 soles, but I got 100, for doing nothing! 100 soles was… wow! A lot of money! But I wanted to get the same that they got. So, I learned, I came into the place and I distracted the guys while the others entered and stole. Another day, we picked a drugstore, I took my bag and I loaded it by myself. By that time, I was twenty-two.

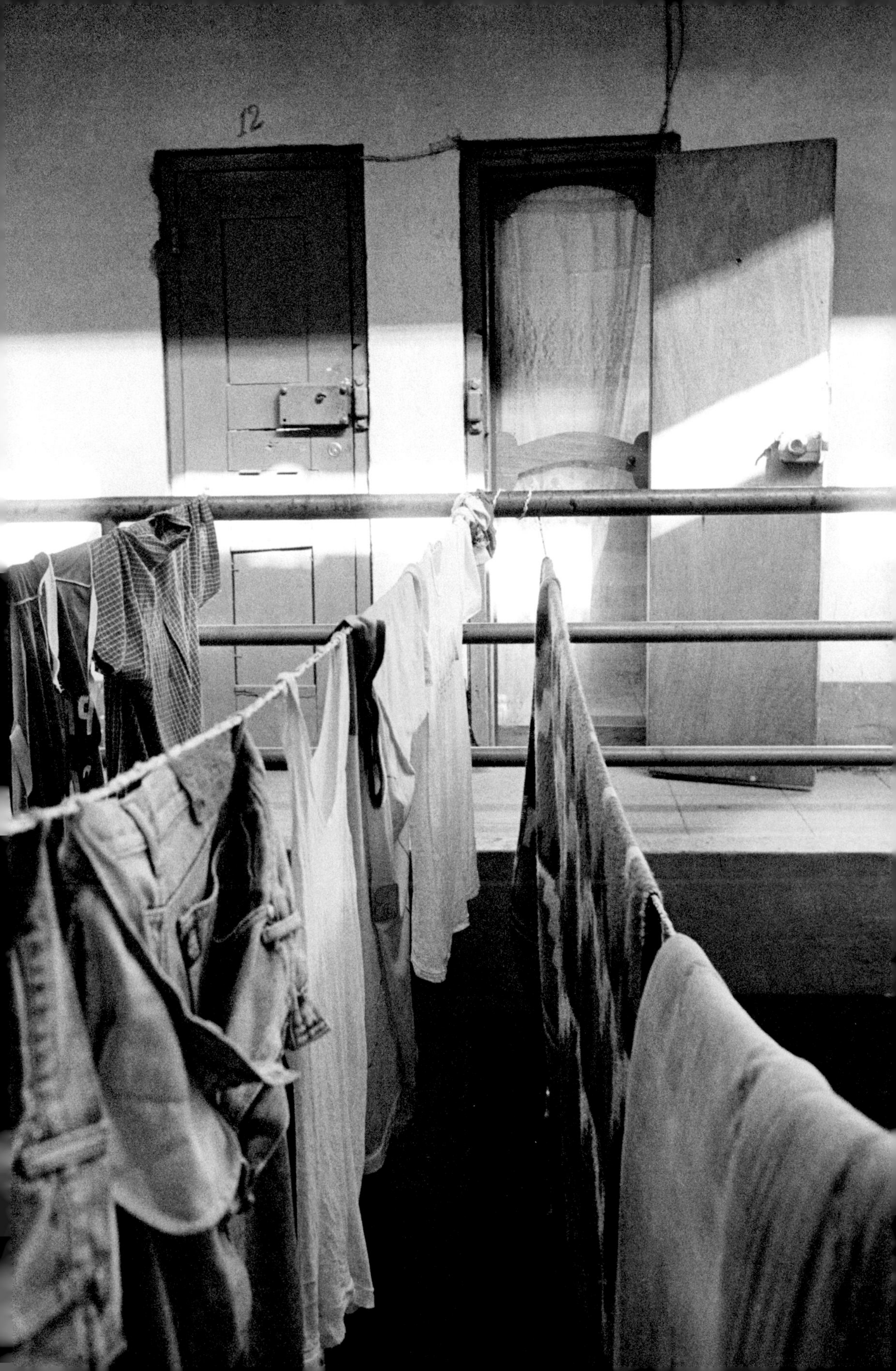

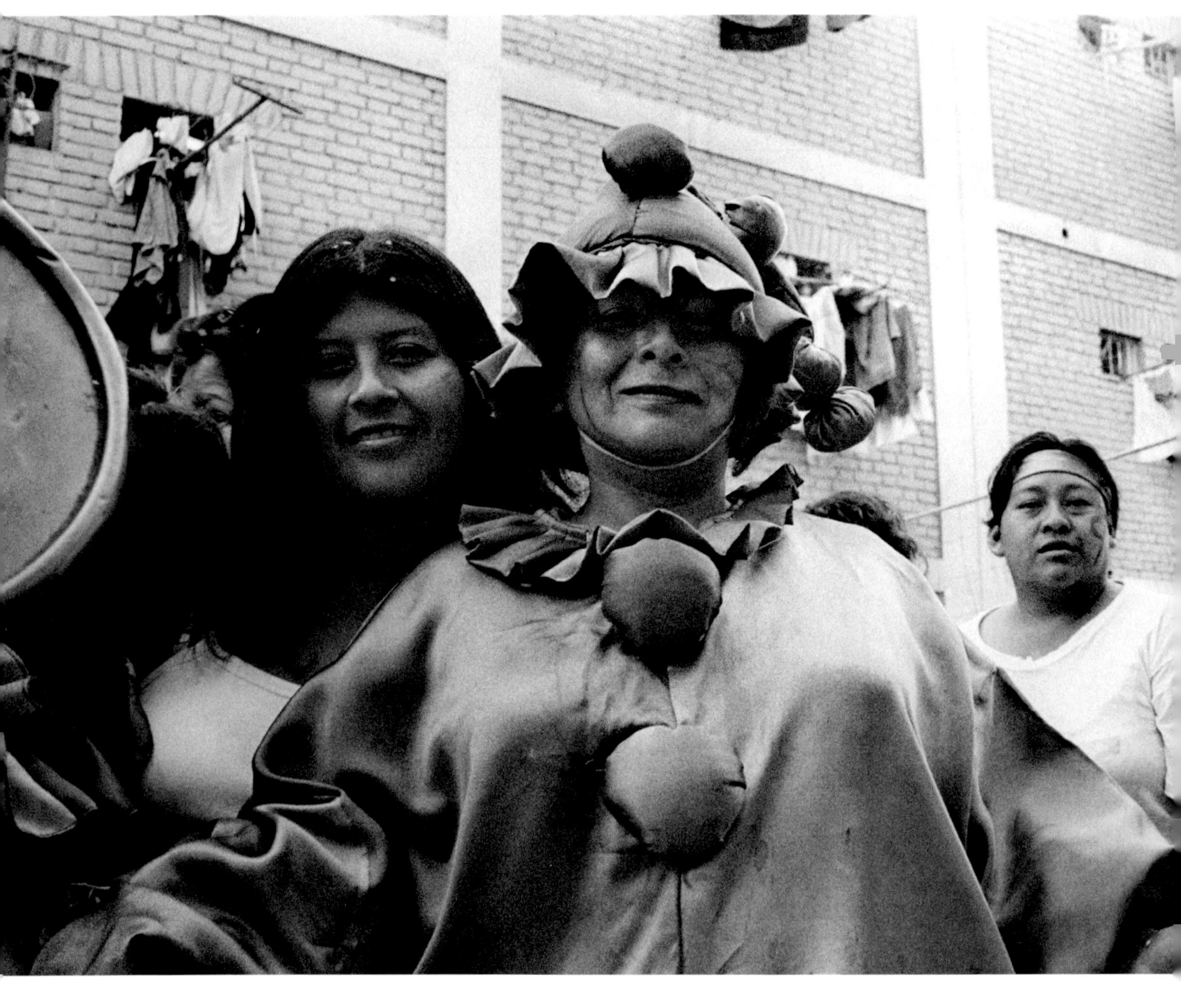

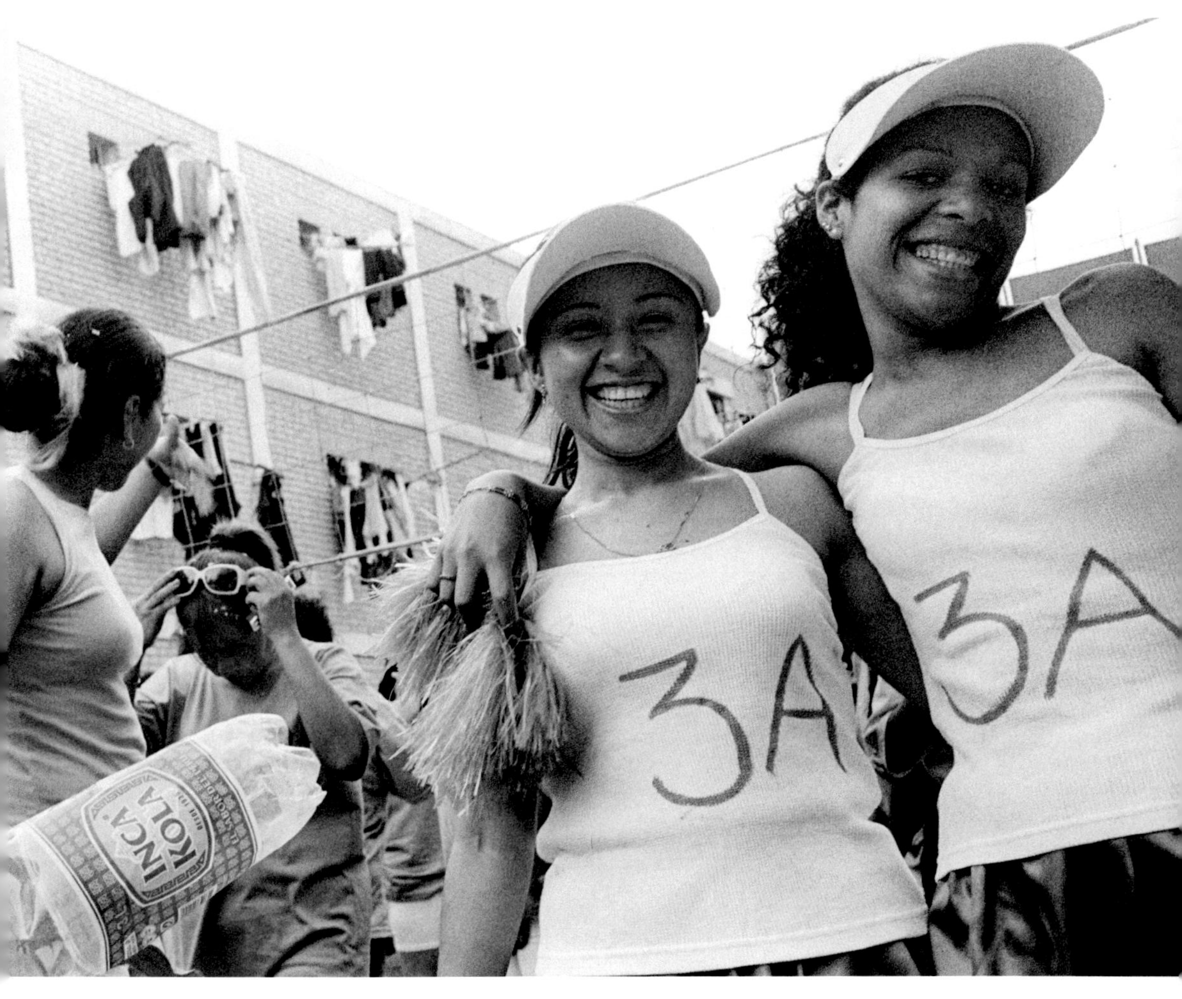

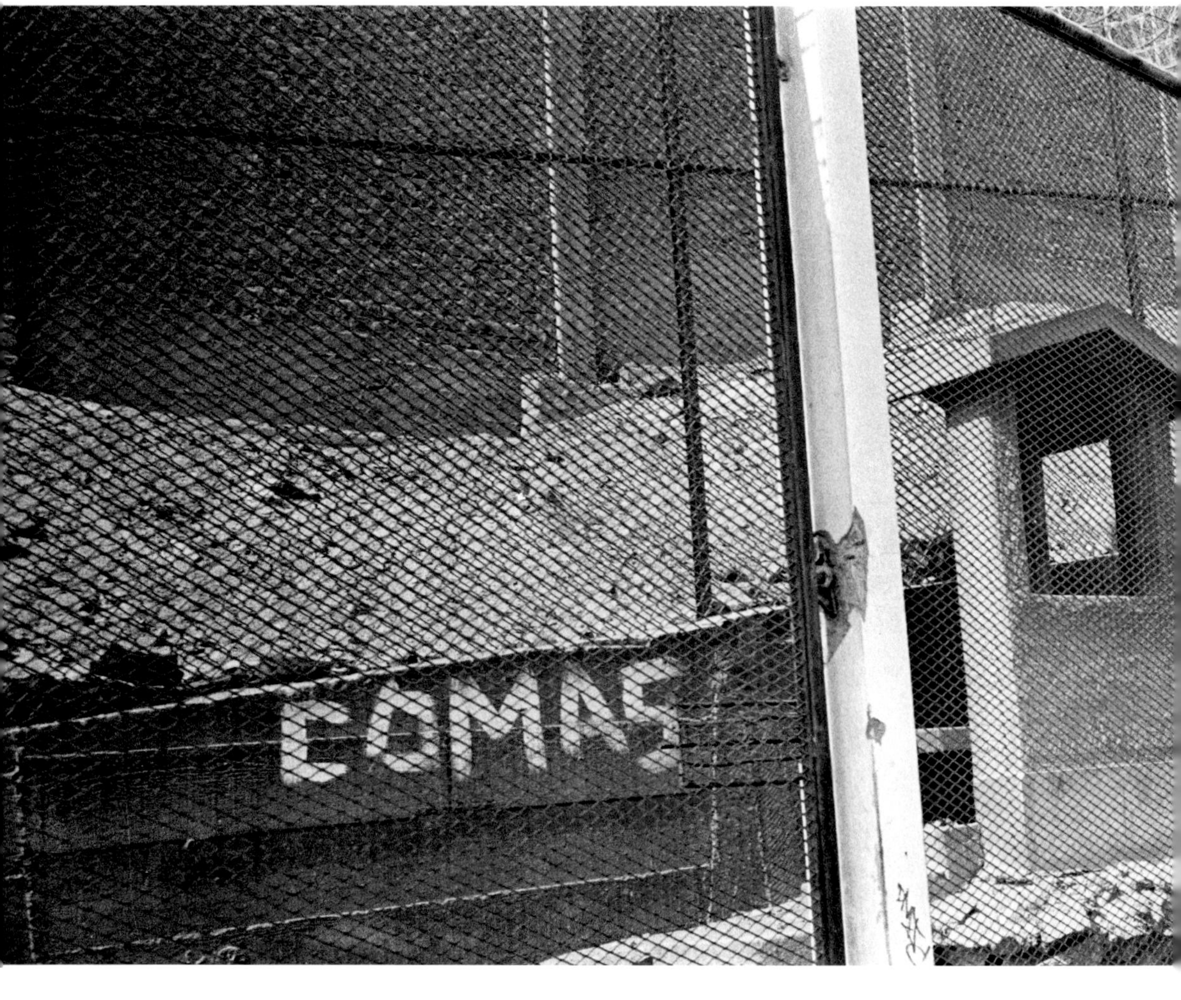
COMAS

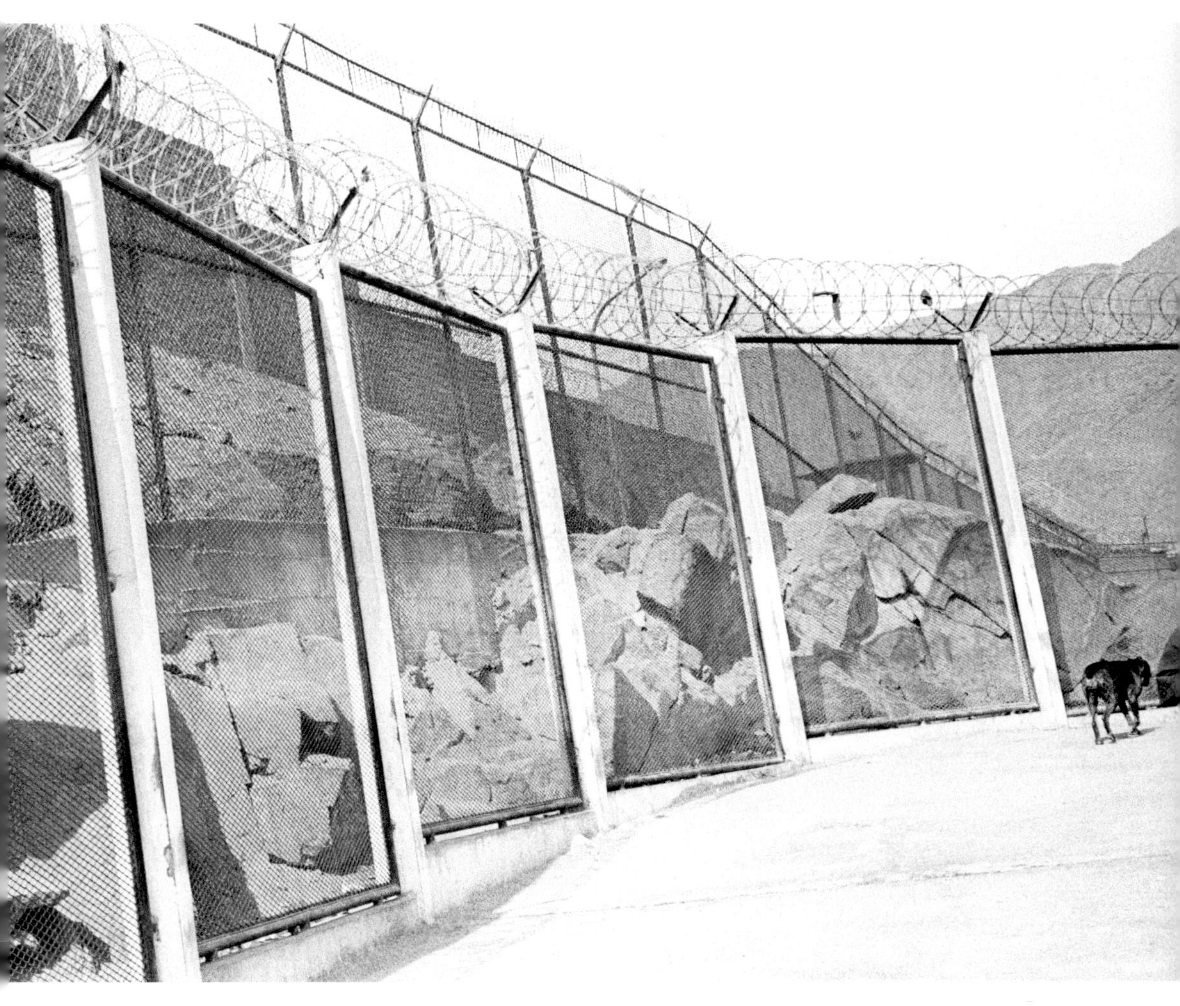

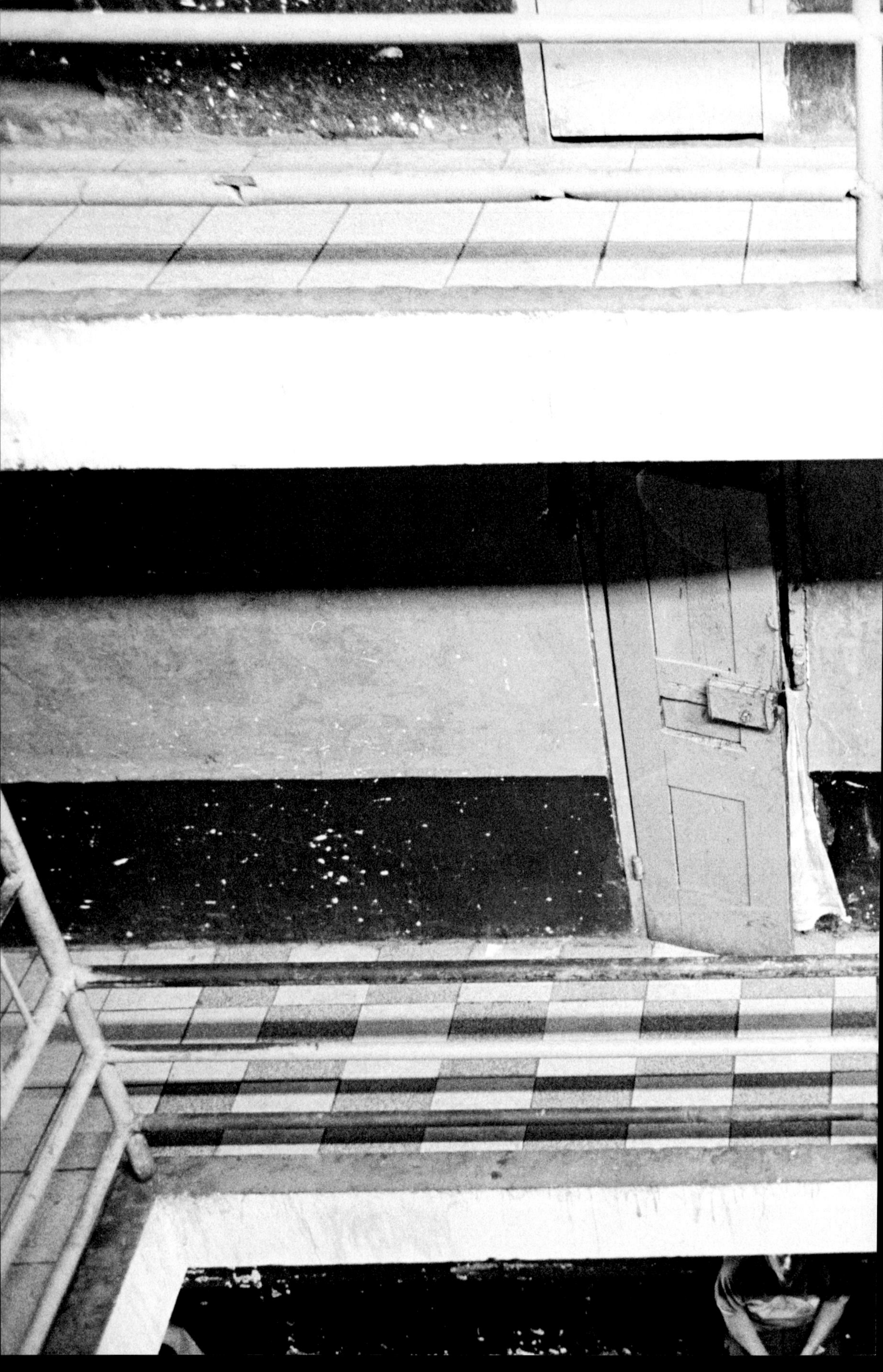

Ivan

43 years old • diagnosed five years ago • Has been in prison since the age of 14

Well, I have seen different attitudes towards people that are carriers. There was a prison block of homosexuals that the people wanted to burn when this disease first appeared. People got infected in the blocks and it was believed that homosexuals had brought it. The minister of justice had to throw them out into the street because the people were going to burn everyone. The reaction was so strong, people didn't know you could also get infected through blood in the needles, and not just homosexuals. There was a block that the whole population of the prison went there to kill. Well, and other things, you know here in Lurigancho life is not worth a thing, people kill each other over a piece of bread.

Sometimes people don't want to touch me because they're afraid of getting infected. This makes me feel like when you offer your friendship as an ordinary human being and they suddenly reject you. But I have never denied I have HIV. I always tell people, I never deny it, rather I help them and I explain to them not to sell their condoms and that even smoking joints we can get infected from bleeding tooth decay. I try to explain about the disease, what I feel so they can help other people, the thing is not if I have it now I will infect other people, I have to take care of myself because of the children, they are the future. Let's say a drop of blood falls on the floor and a little kid comes, you know, children play and if they come across the blood, they can get infected. It's the babies we have to take care of the most.

Well, now I want to start preaching the Word and if it is possible to come out of here alive, because I will be out in a year and a half, I hope the Lord keeps me alive.

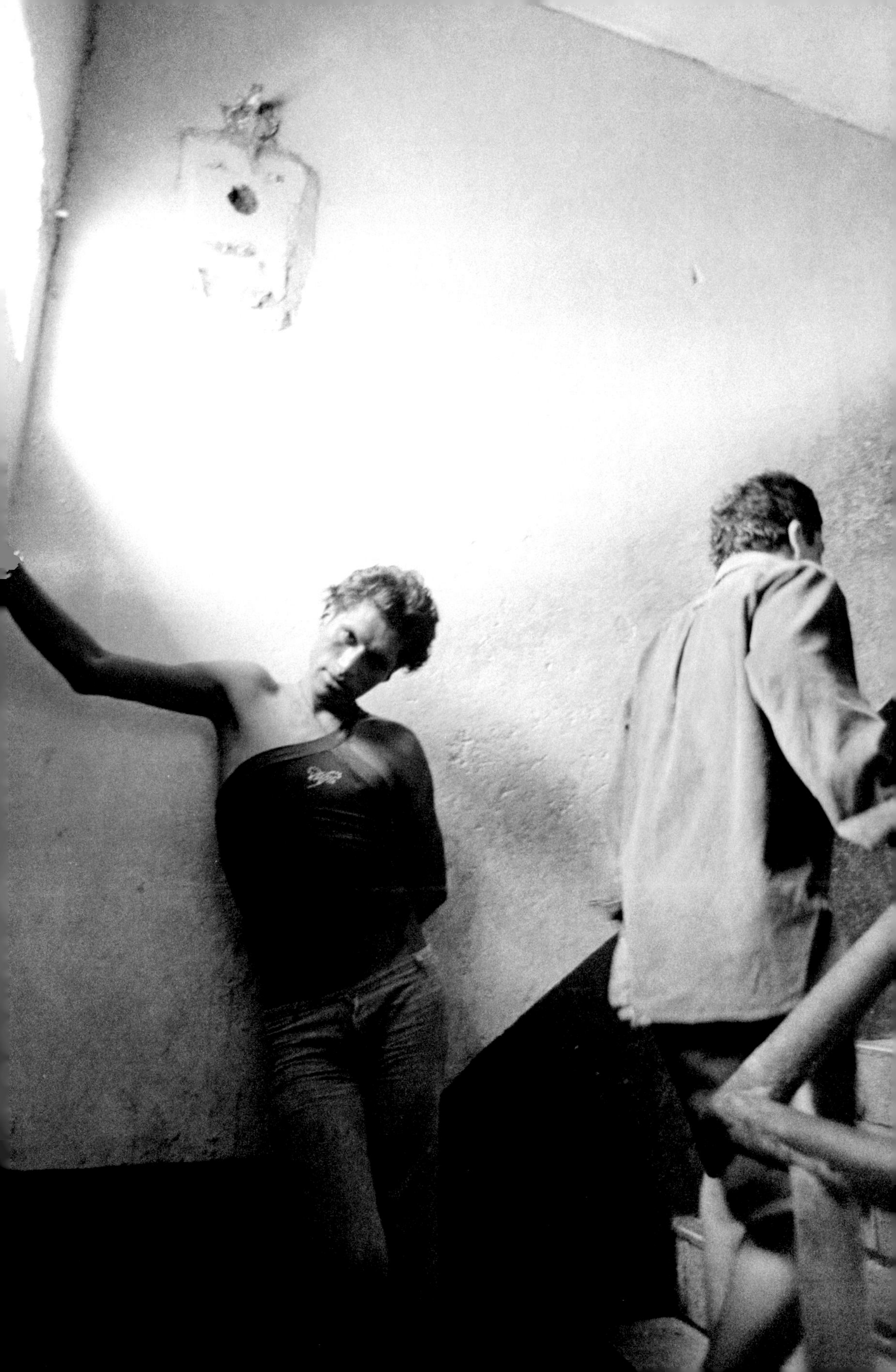

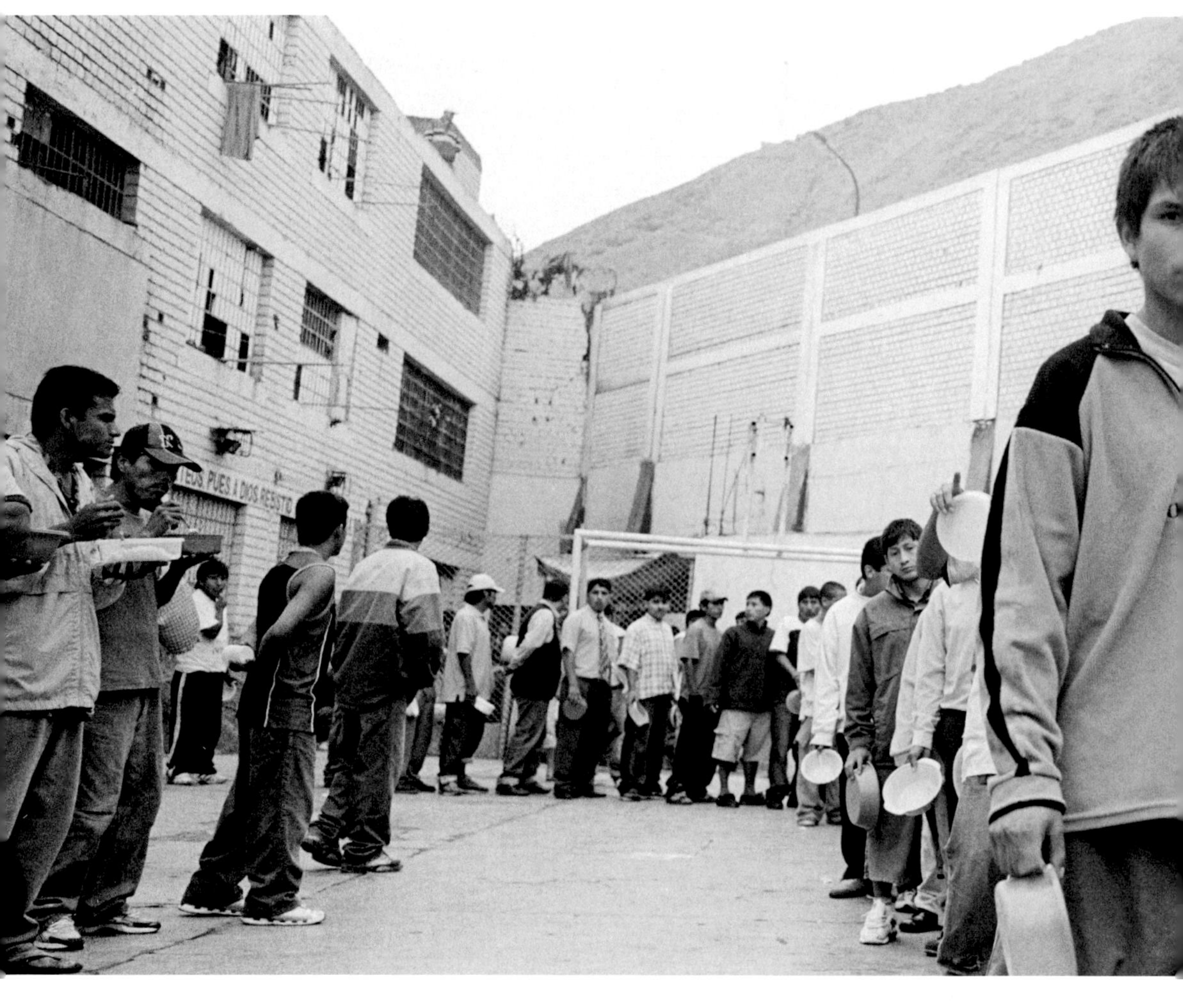

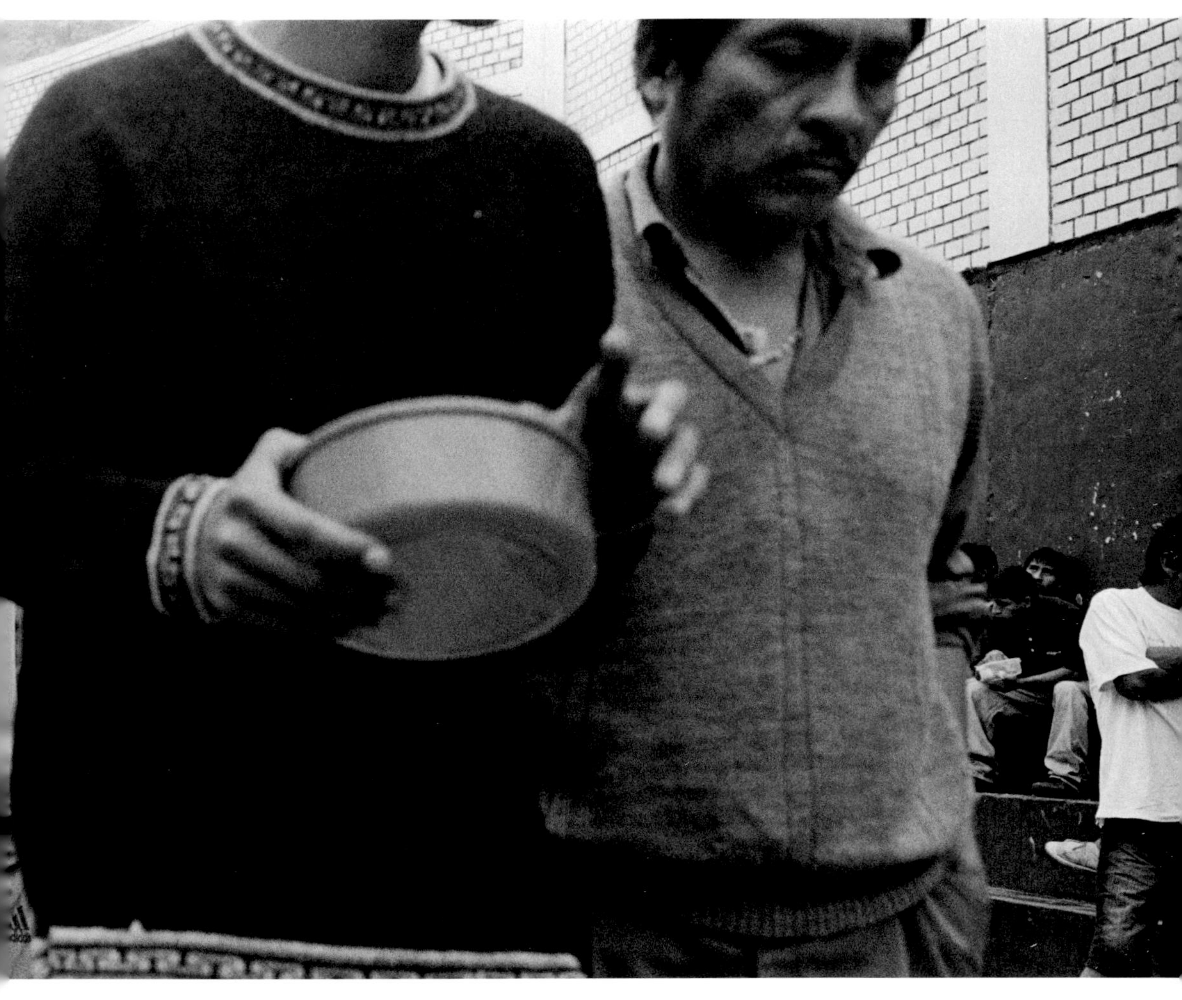

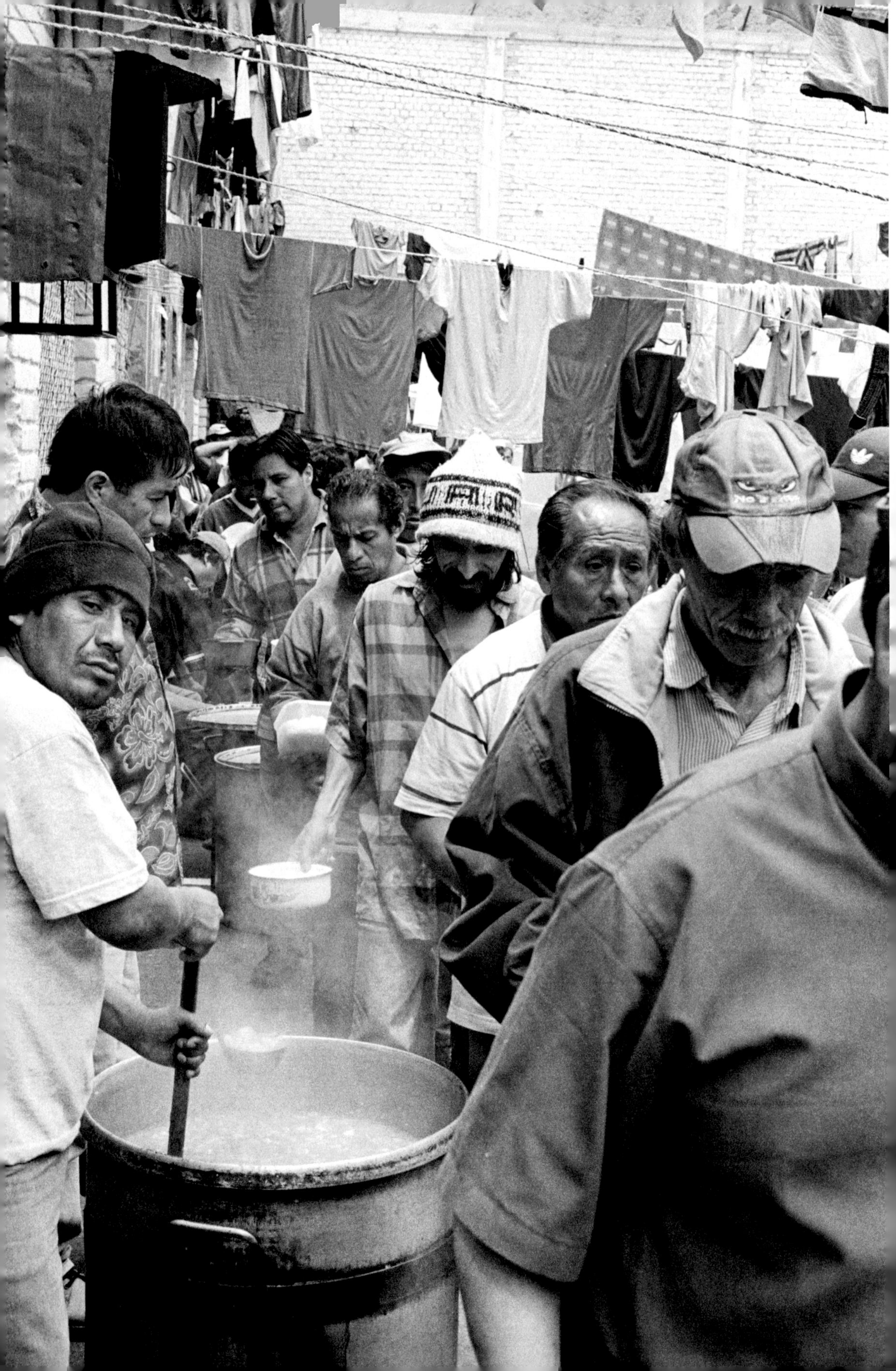

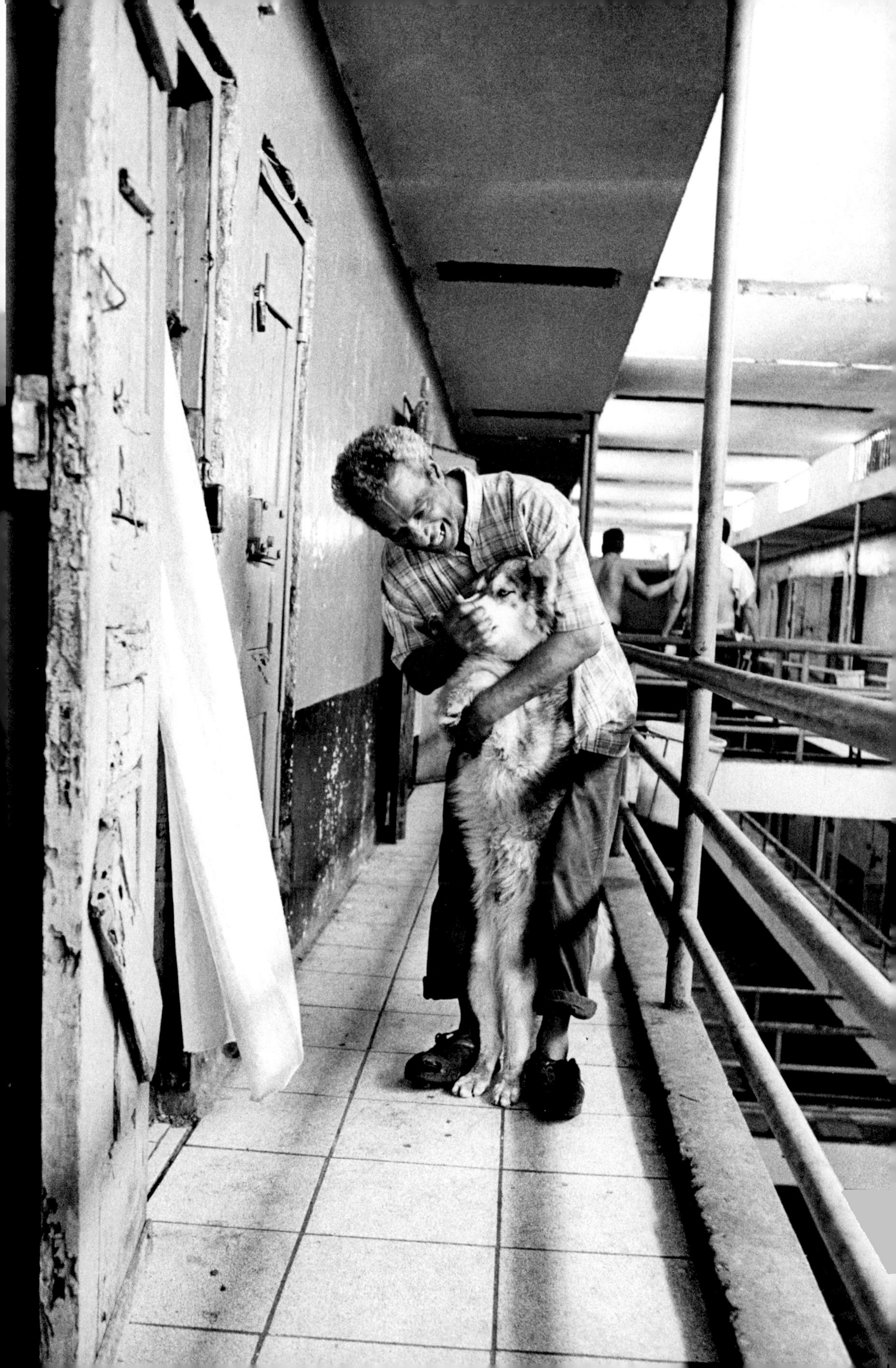

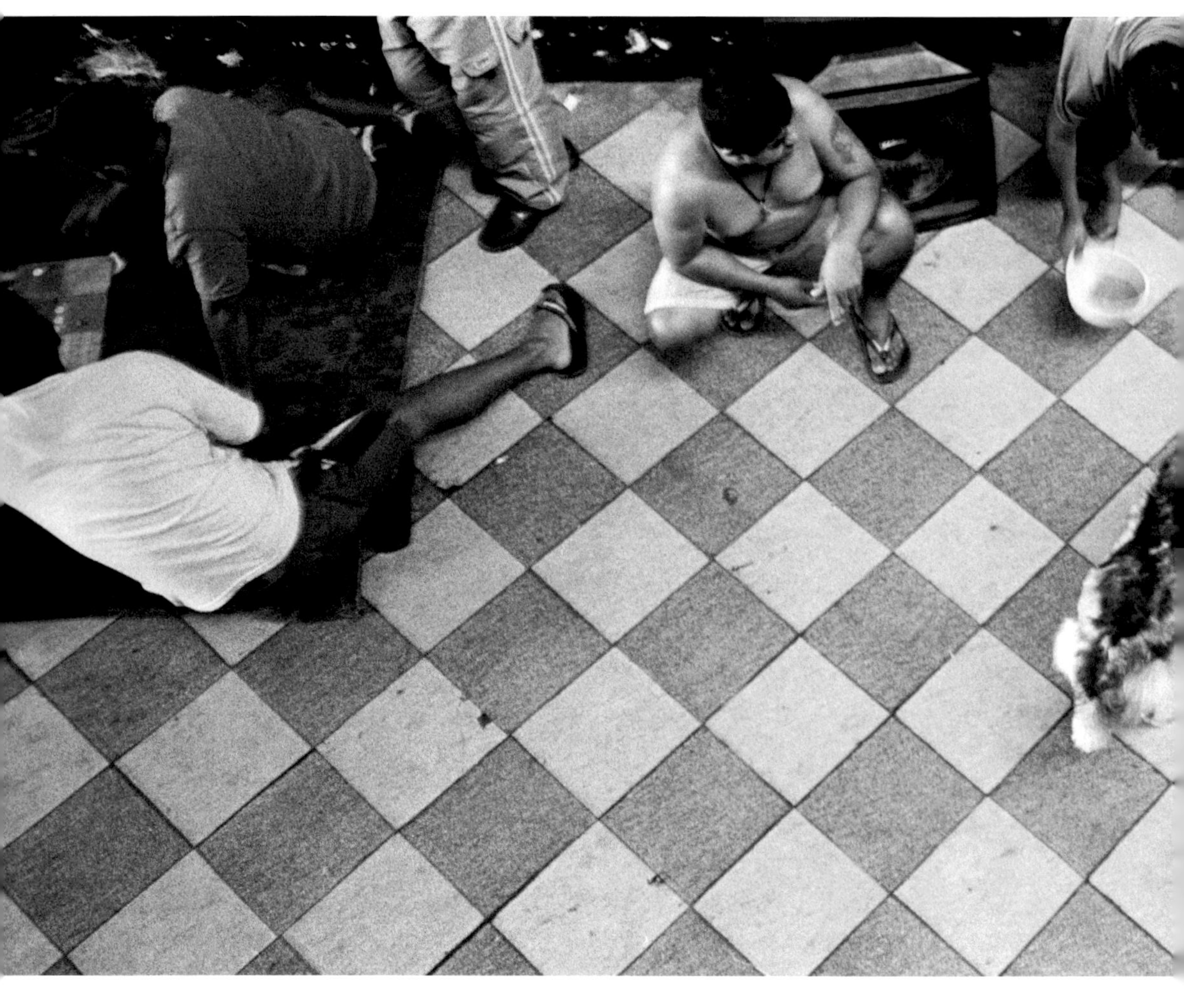

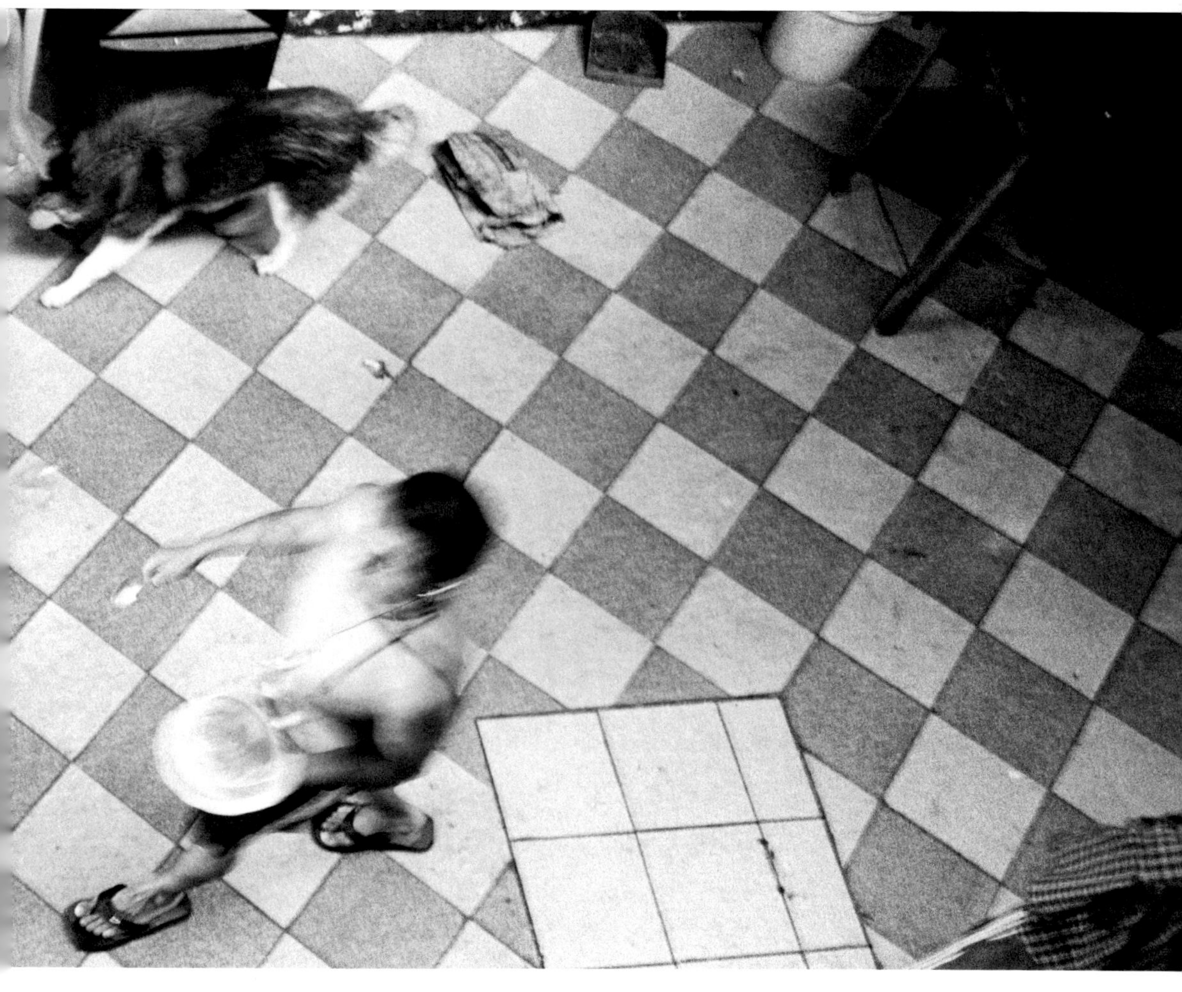

LUIS ALBERTO

**42 YEARS OLD • THREE YEARS SPENT IN LURIGANCHO PRISON
DIAGNOSED ON FEBRUARY 22, 2005**

Before my diagnosis, I had no information. I had only heard about AIDS and saw how people died from this disease. I watched my friends die but I almost never got near them.

No, I never thought I would get infected, for me it is a simple disease, that is, I have learned to live with it. At first, it is a shock, it seems you are going to die every single day, for you it's a day less, but thanks to God and science you learn how to live with the disease and manage. I am thankful to all the counselors here and to Médecins Sans Frontières, most of all because the workshops helped me a lot, of course if they hadn't been able to continue here, I would have given up.

At present, I consider myself just like the others but of course there are one or two that spit at you because you have AIDS. I don't pay attention nowadays, but in the first period it really hurt me.

Yes, after I was diagnosed my life changed in relation to what it was before... At least I didn't used to love myself much, I was always drinking, getting high. I hurt my family most of all, I didn't rob them or anything but I ran away from home; I was never home, I mostly lived with friends selling drugs. But now my life has changed a lot because I have learned to appreciate my family, at least where I am now, no one comes to see me, just my family, they are the ones that are there for me. Likewise, I have learned to love myself, I am more calm, I have learned to appreciate things, not to criticize people, because before, I used to complain, I wouldn't go near them (those with HIV), I was very frightened of those people. I was very frightened of people with tuberculosis, I wouldn't even go near them. On the contrary, now I live with them, and this has sunk deep and that is how I will be when I get out.

Of course I have seen marginalization. For example, towards me, I wanted to work in the kitchen and they told me no because of the gossip that I could cut myself and they would get infected. They stopped me right there and then - they don't want to share your spoon, even though it is not contagious. Sometimes they want to cut themselves off from you but as one who has already learned to live, you don't care what they think. If they do think that, I think they are mistaken and that this is due to their ignorance. If they went to workshops on all these diseases like our families do, I think they wouldn't treat us like this, and sometimes it hurts, but what are we to do? We won't get worked up about nothing either, we have to go forward that's all. I think they should receive guidance so they can learn to put up with the people that are sick. But there are some people that have not gone to the workshops but know how to understand you quite well. Also, the health delegate calls me and asks me to wash his clothes, he helps me pay for my food and one thing or another and there are a lot of people like him, but as there are other people who reject you, you have to learn to live here.

All of my family knows about my diagnosis, really, my brothers love me very much, they are there for me throughout everything, it was easy to tell them because we were brought up as a close family. Of course they suffered a lot at the beginning but I had to give them courage myself, I cannot be whining or crying because I am the patient and when they leave they suffer. At first I didn't notice, but little by little I have learned. Sometimes I don't feel so well but I hold on and it goes away and they go home feeling happy. I also have to help them to overcome the problem.

Well, people do not take their medicines because of drugs and alcohol, that is the main reason alongside family abandonment, because here when the family abandons you, what does the person do? He finds refuge in a glass of alcohol or in drugs, and that is the main problem. What I'm saying is they are not interested because truth be told, drugs help you, and truth be told, you are in a kind of sickness and it keeps you up, but if you stop taking drugs, you will find yourself down on the floor, that is the main reason.

I hope to go out to work and show my family what I never was able to give them before. That is what I want to do because my life has changed and I want to work and have a family outside, and leave my past buried in prison.

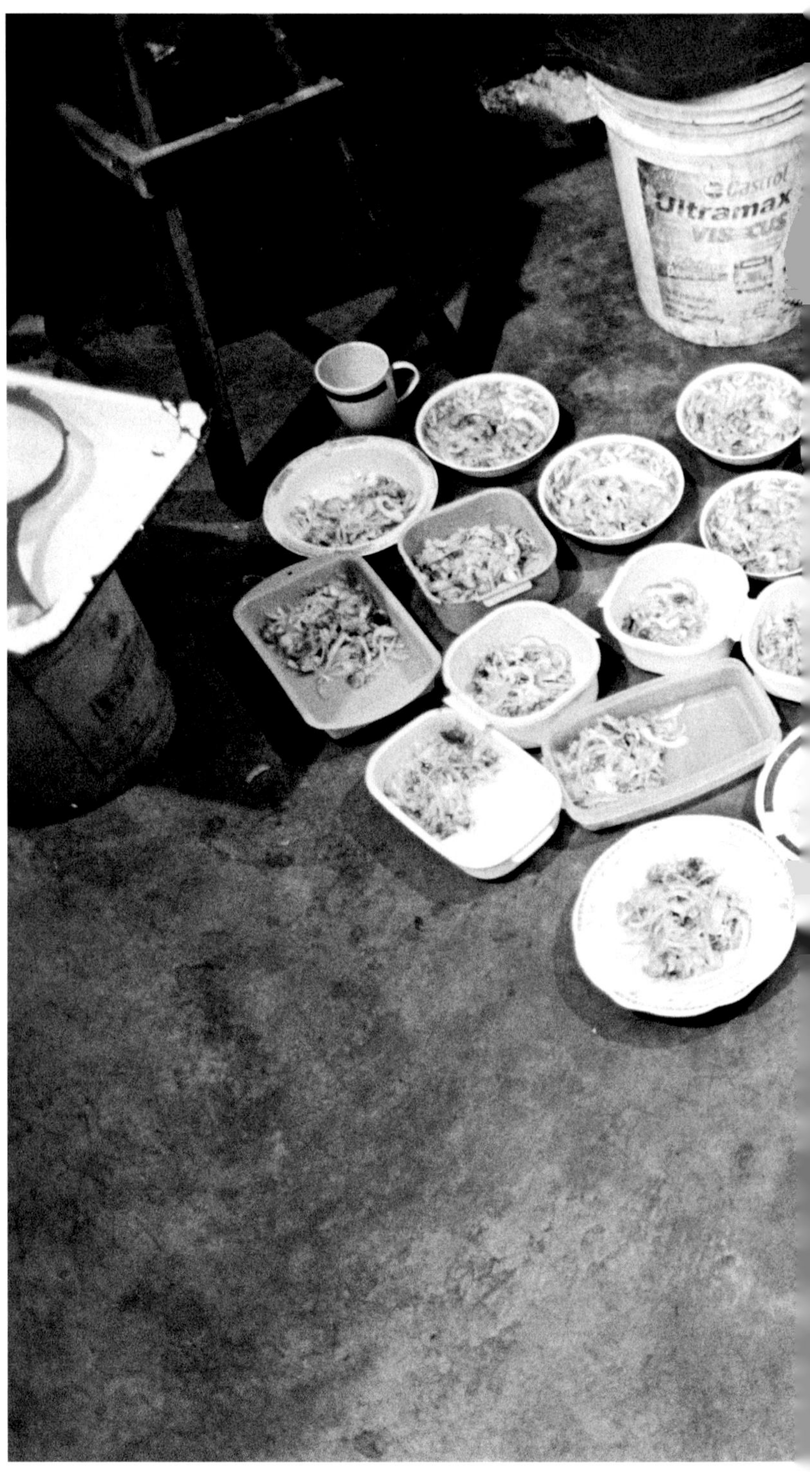

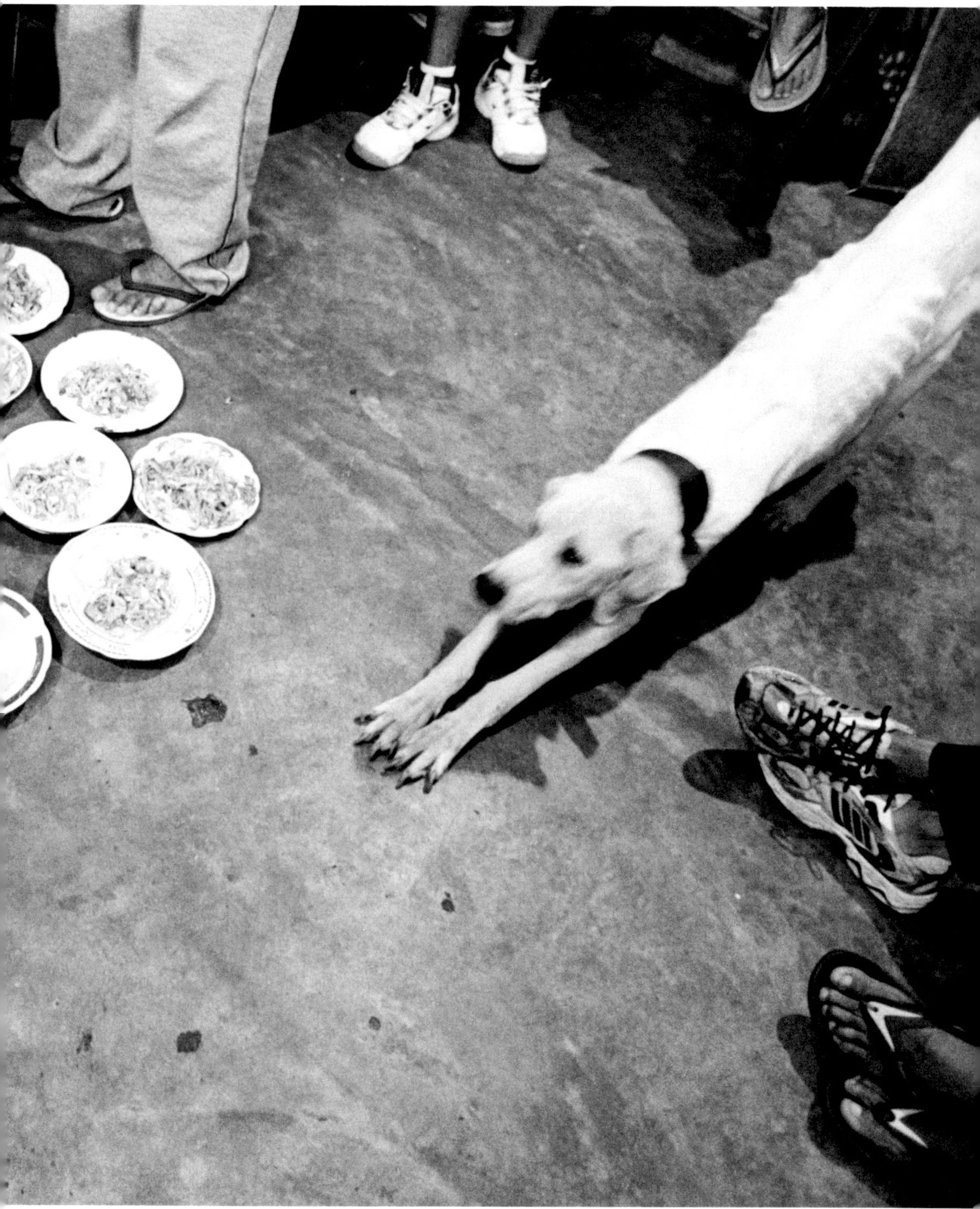

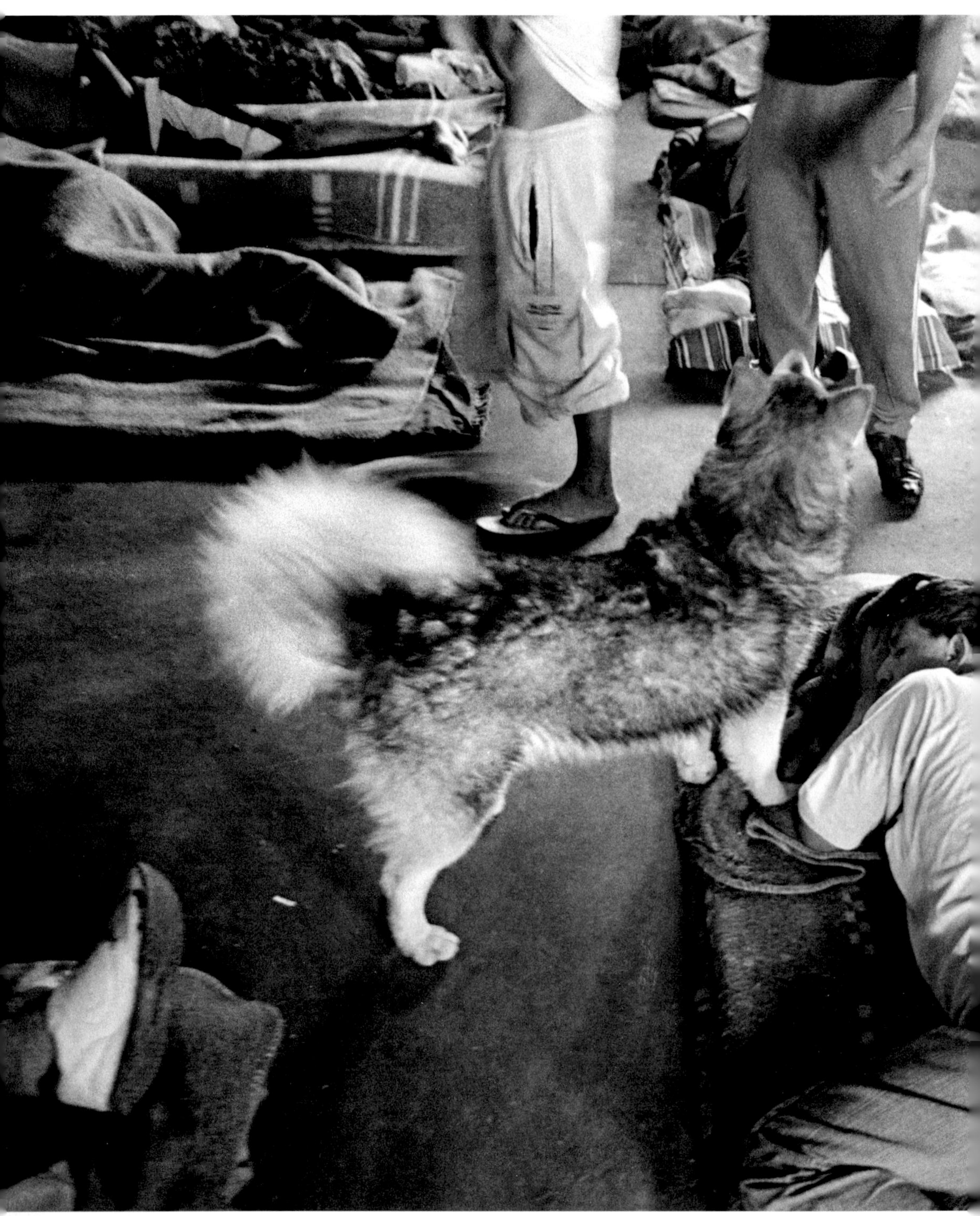

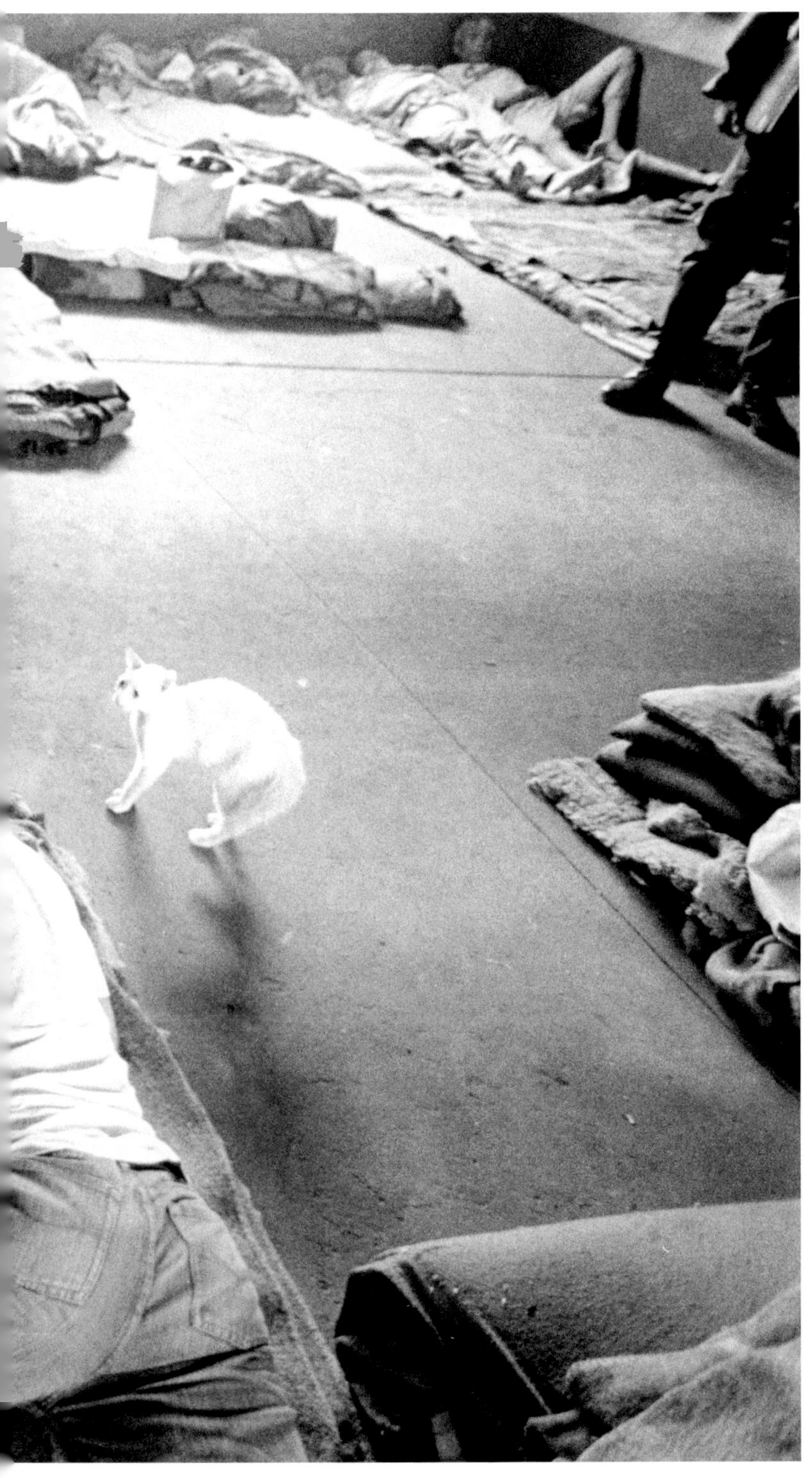

MIGUEL

31 YEARS OLD

I am 31 years old, they diagnosed me outside, but I didn't give it much importance. I remember I went to the Dos de Mayo Hospital where they treated me badly, as I didn't have any references like here in prison, where I have had lectures and have acquired knowledge about the disease; so I got depressed and never had treatment. I ignored it all and my ulcer got bad, I had gastritis but I didn't pay it much attention until one day I got really sick.

It is very important to be well-informed because you learn to live with this disease and learn to follow your treatment correctly. Each day you find out about more things and about medicines or what is good for herpes.

Before all of this, I used to think that this was a mortal disease, that it killed you and that there never was going to be a cure for it. It was a disease, how do you say, like a punishment from God to people, and that you would get infected and that in a week or a month you would die, or that's what I thought.

Yes, at one point I thought I could be infected because I lived a very irresponsible life. I practically did not have a full childhood since I lost my mother when I was 8, and I began to hang out with older people and grew up quickly. At twelve I already knew the whorehouses, I drank, I had countless sexual relationships with whores or with homosexuals or transvestites, until this disease hit me, but I thought that I would never, ever get this disease.

Unfortunately, I was wrong and I learned to get over it and now I don't care if they insult me or don't insult me, what I'm interested in is in living, for my children, my wife and for life itself. Now this is not a disease, it is an infection, and before everybody used to die but now there is something that can block the virus, the retrovirus.

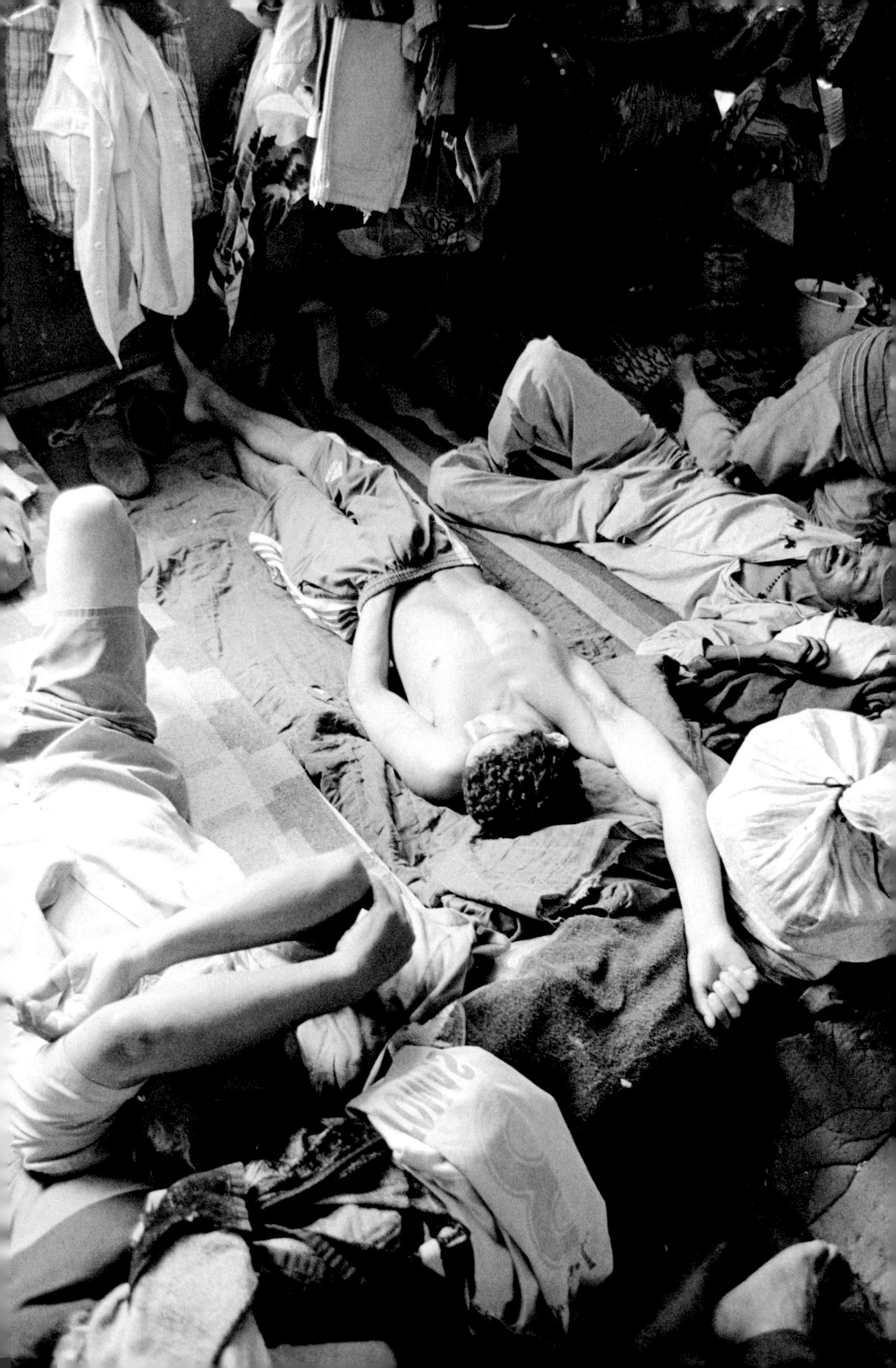

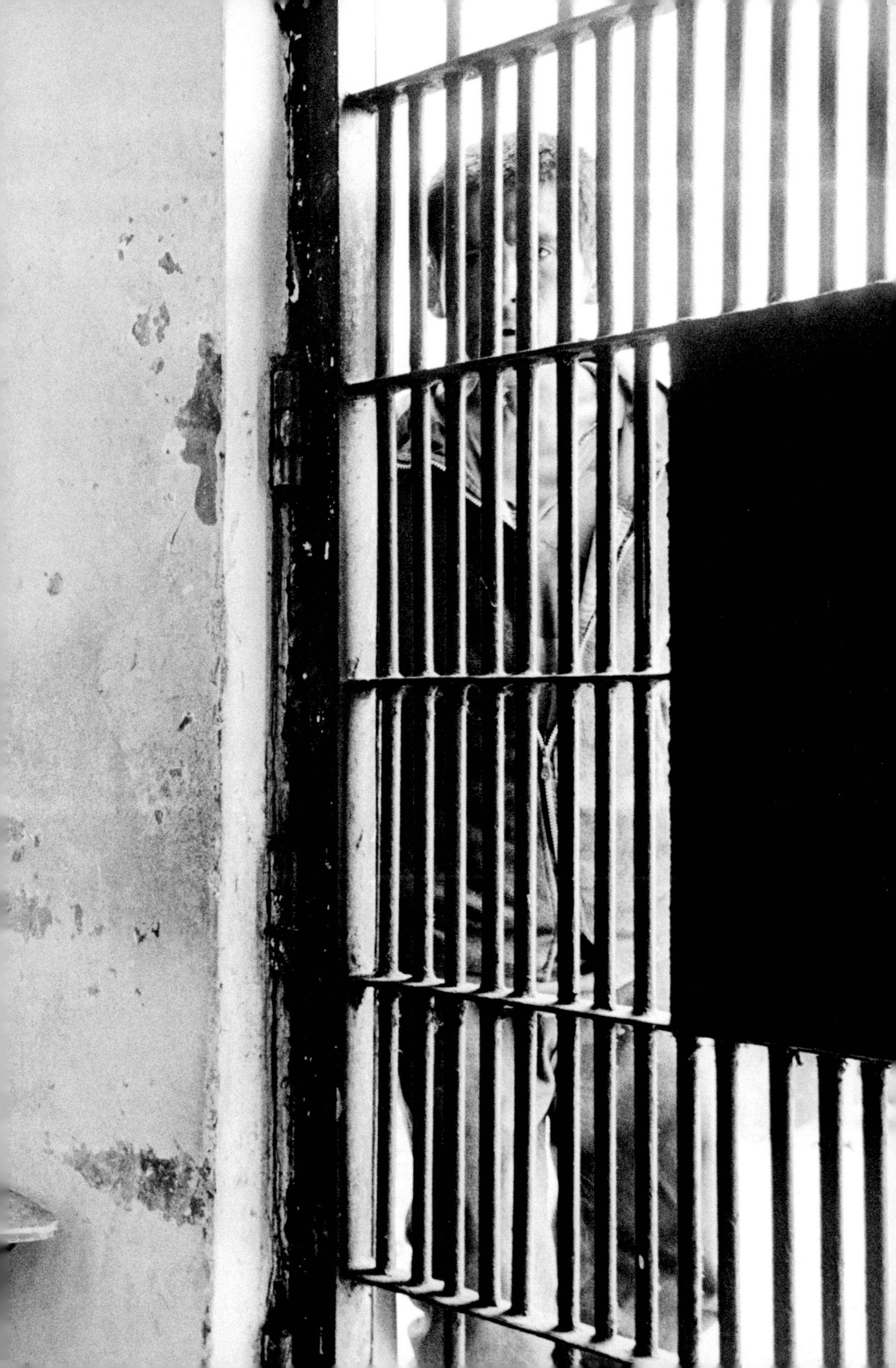

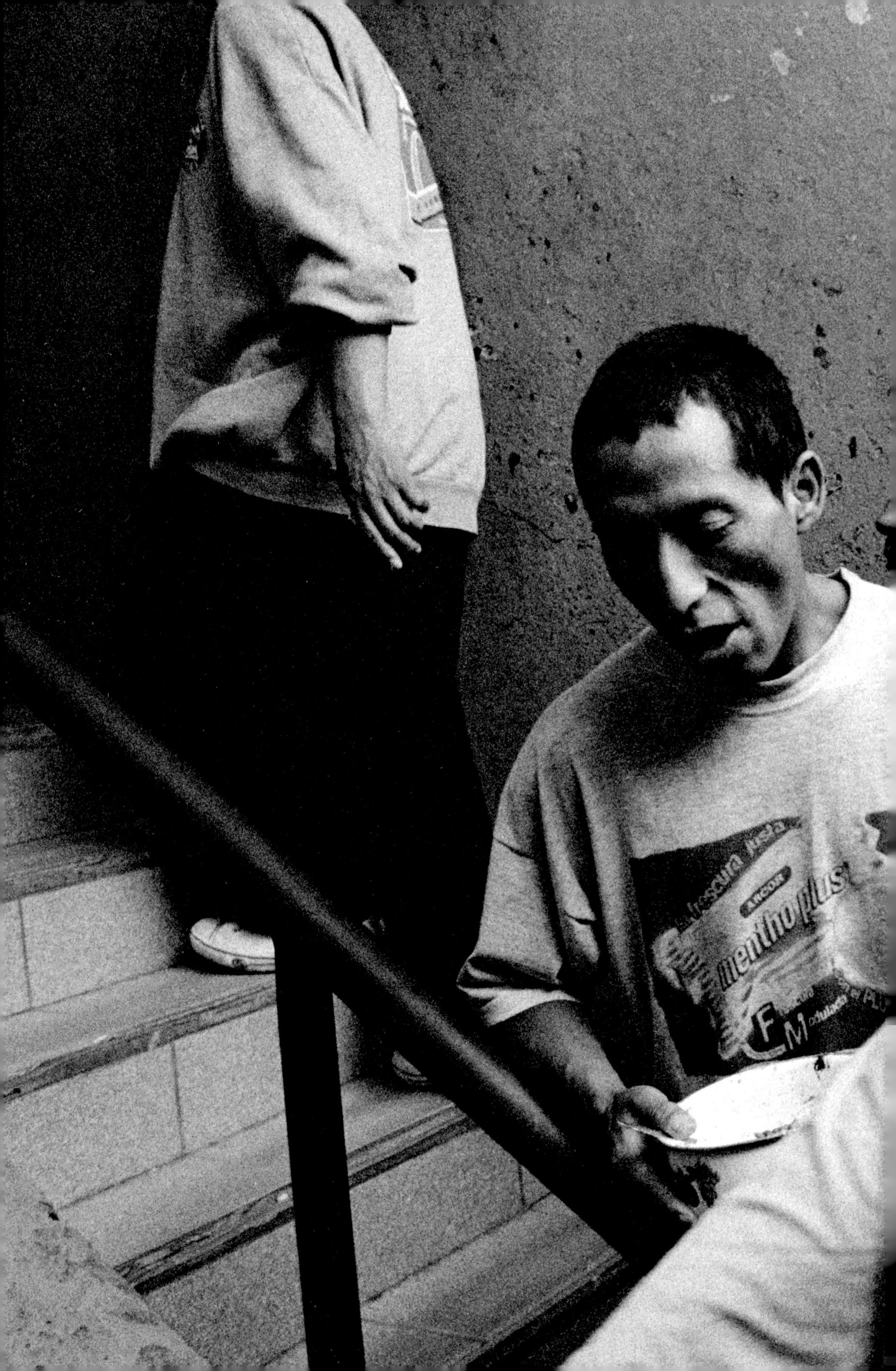

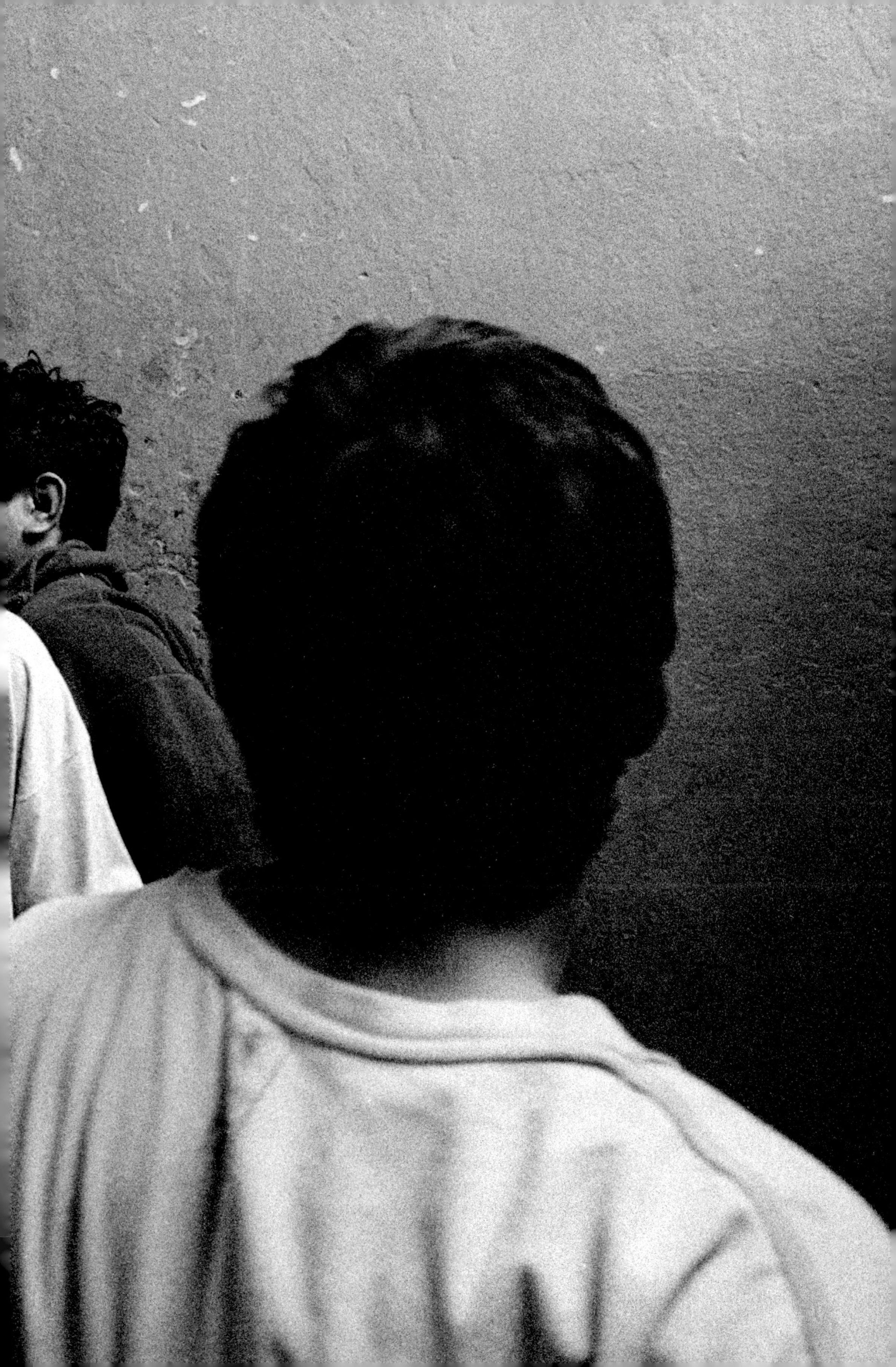

WONDER WOMAN

**27 YEARS OLD, TRANSVESTITE • HAS BEEN IN LURIGANCHO PRISON FOR 6 YEARS
WONDER WOMAN IS AN ALIAS USED TO PROTECT HIS IDENTITY**

I don't remember how I ended up in the "Hole", maybe they got me drunk, and I got mouthy with a guard - the chato (short guy) got offended and sent me to the Británico, that's what they also call the "Hole", I don't know why. I gave some money to the policeman in charge so he could put me in a nice cell. But then as others also gave him money, he took me out again.

I didn't want to go to sleep, but he forced me out, grabbed me, opened the lock and took me out of the cell I had paid for. In the 'Hole' they asked me to have sex with them, I said "No, no, no, I don't want to do anything", then I started to cry. They couldn't stand my tears, one day they tried to cut me with a spoon and forced me to have sex with all of them, with all. Of course, everything was with a condom, they even called out to the policeman, "Hey policeman, a condom, hey policeman a condom!", and the policeman went and brought condoms and sold

them to them. I didn't want more, sometimes I screamed, but as they were all high I had to give in, because maybe in their insanity they might do something to me. Then I pretended to be humble because I was afraid. Anything to get out of the "Hole."

Then I almost lost my mind because I became sick from alcohol and drugs. My wounds got infected, it looked like they had burned me. A boil developed from my stomach to my side. All my back was bitten, my silicone got infected, I was in a very bad state and they sent me to the doctor's office. I was at last able to get out of there. They gave me a shot and my boil healed and I got well. Luckily, it was not serious, as I thought it might have been a venereal disease.

Now I am well, thanks to Sarita Colonia (the inmates are her devotees. She is believed be a miracle worker, born in the 1940s). I have my partner, I take care of him but he doesn't want anybody to know I am with him because they will think he is a maricón (homosexual), and even more so if they know I have AIDS. Here, they beat us up for that, "Sidosos!" (a person with AIDS) they yell at us. We keep quiet to avoid being mistreated.

Sometimes at night I think about the cells at the 'Hole'. The eight cells, where there were from 15 to 20 people. Imagine what it was like at breakfast, lunch or dinner time, because to be honest, we always had food. There were also drugs. Sometimes to buy drugs, some kids accepted the abuse. They call them caletas (name given to inmates who do not publicly say they are gay). But in my case, due to my sexual condition, they forced me into all those cells. When I remember I really get sicoseado (psychotic). I remember in the last cell there was a boy I knew, he was my friend. There they treated me better, they saw I was sick and they all took care of me. The guys themselves talked to the policeman to let me out, because he didn't want to believe I was sick, until I went to the doctor. Afterwards I was tired, if I didn't accept, they didn't let me sleep, they would pester me.

It's been a year since this happened.

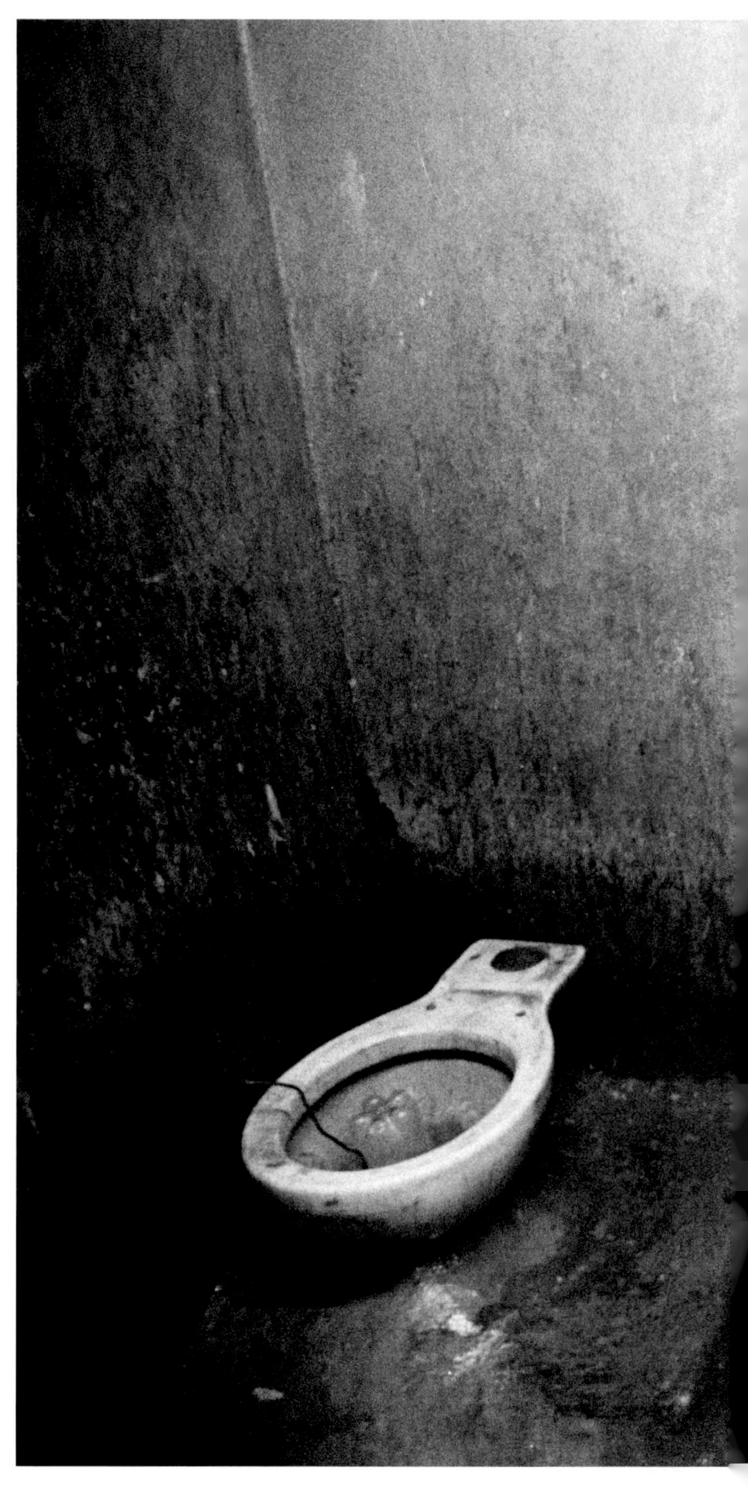

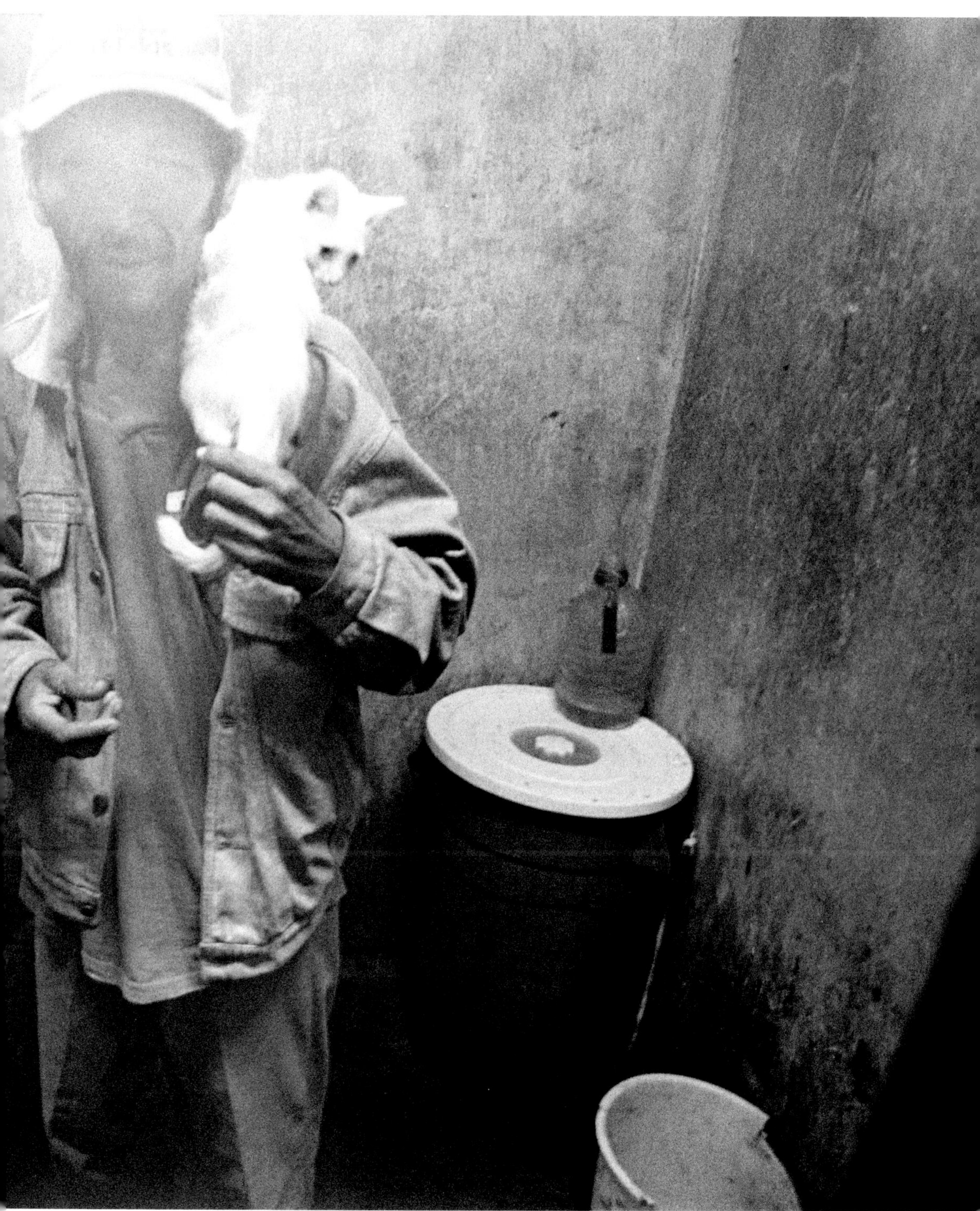

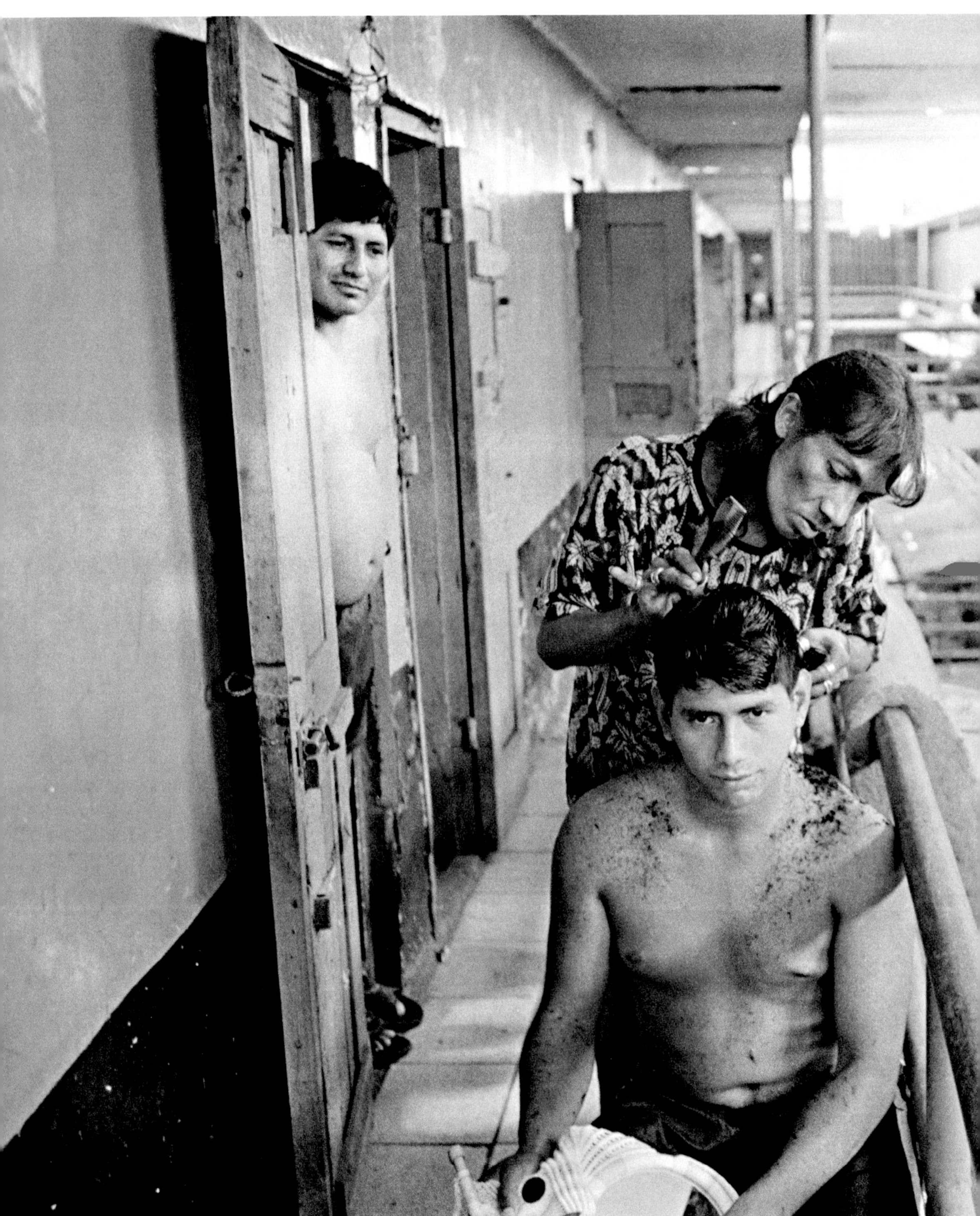

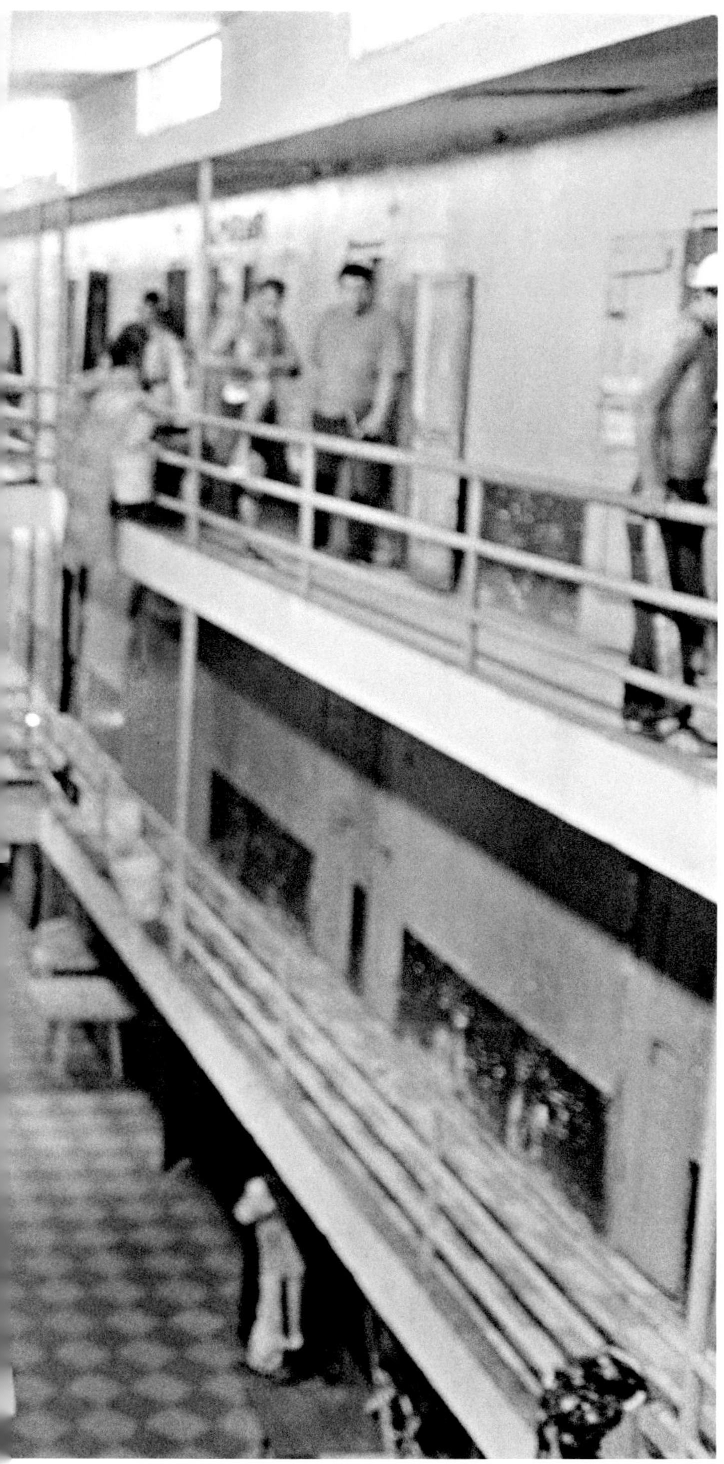

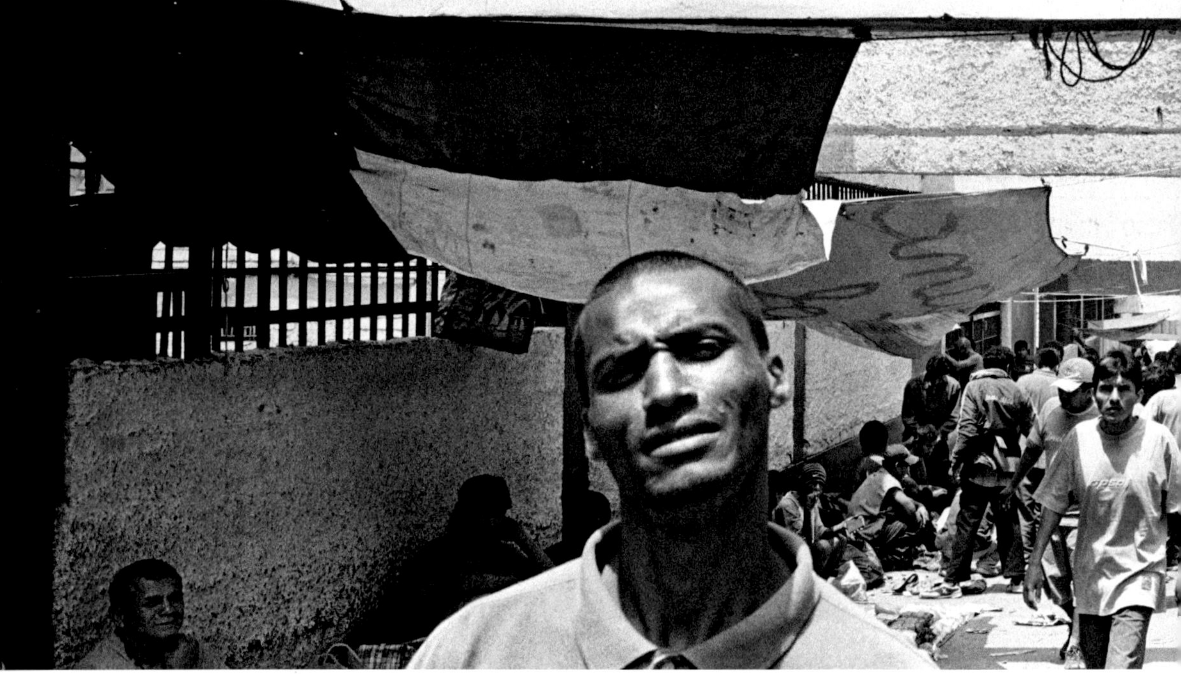
GRACIAS POR
PAB. 6 S.M.P.A

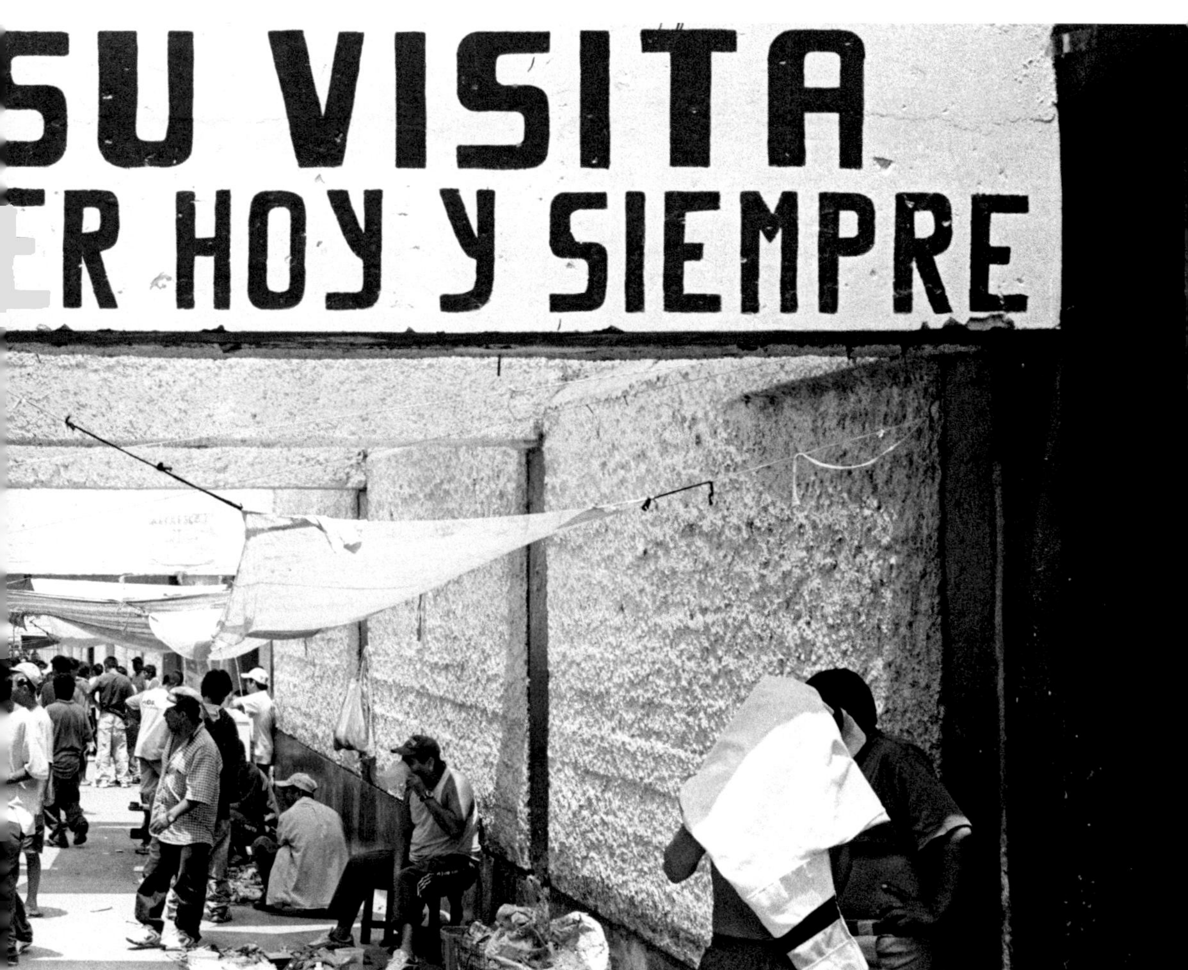

SU VISITA
ER HOY Y SIEMPRE

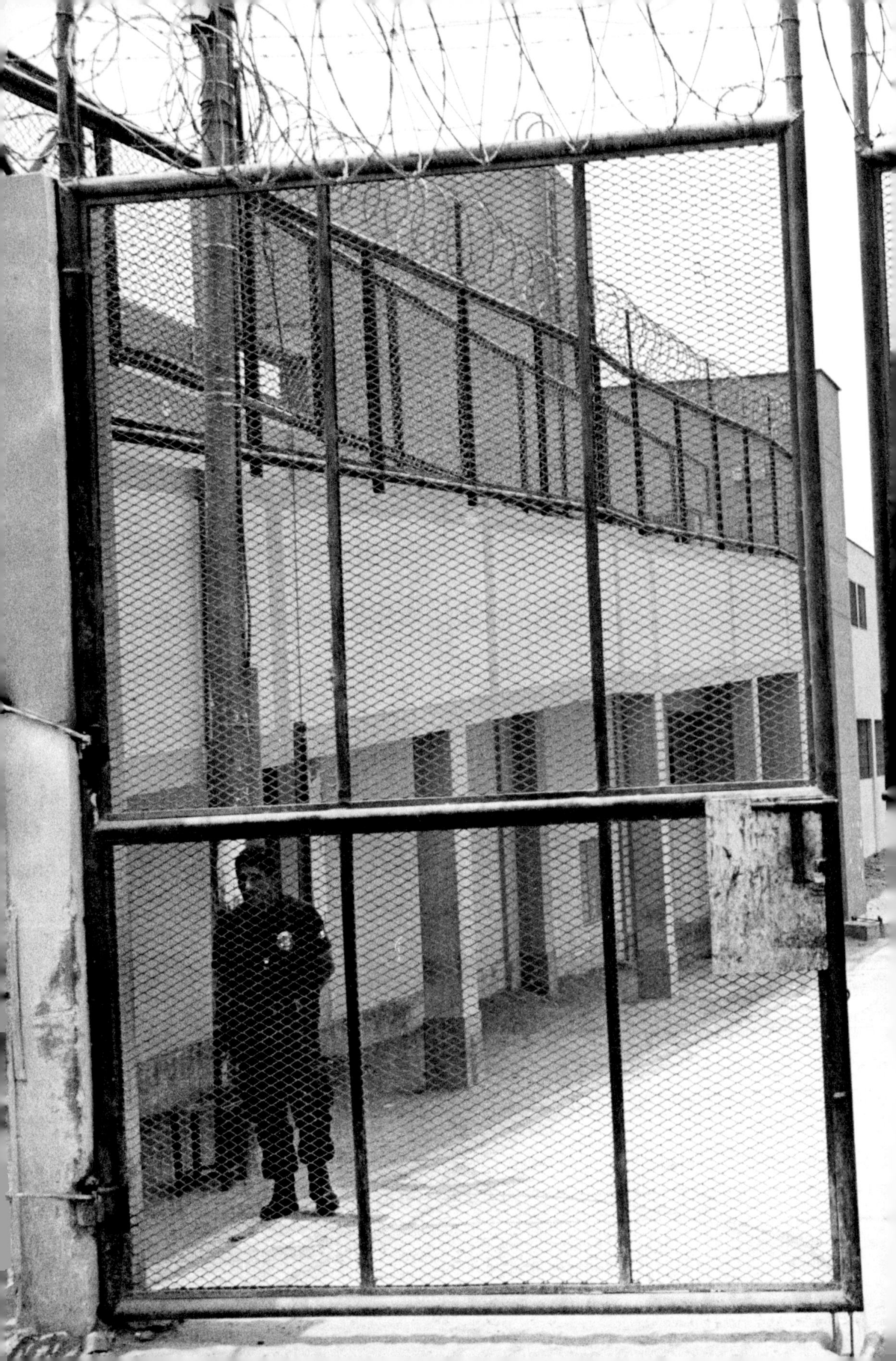

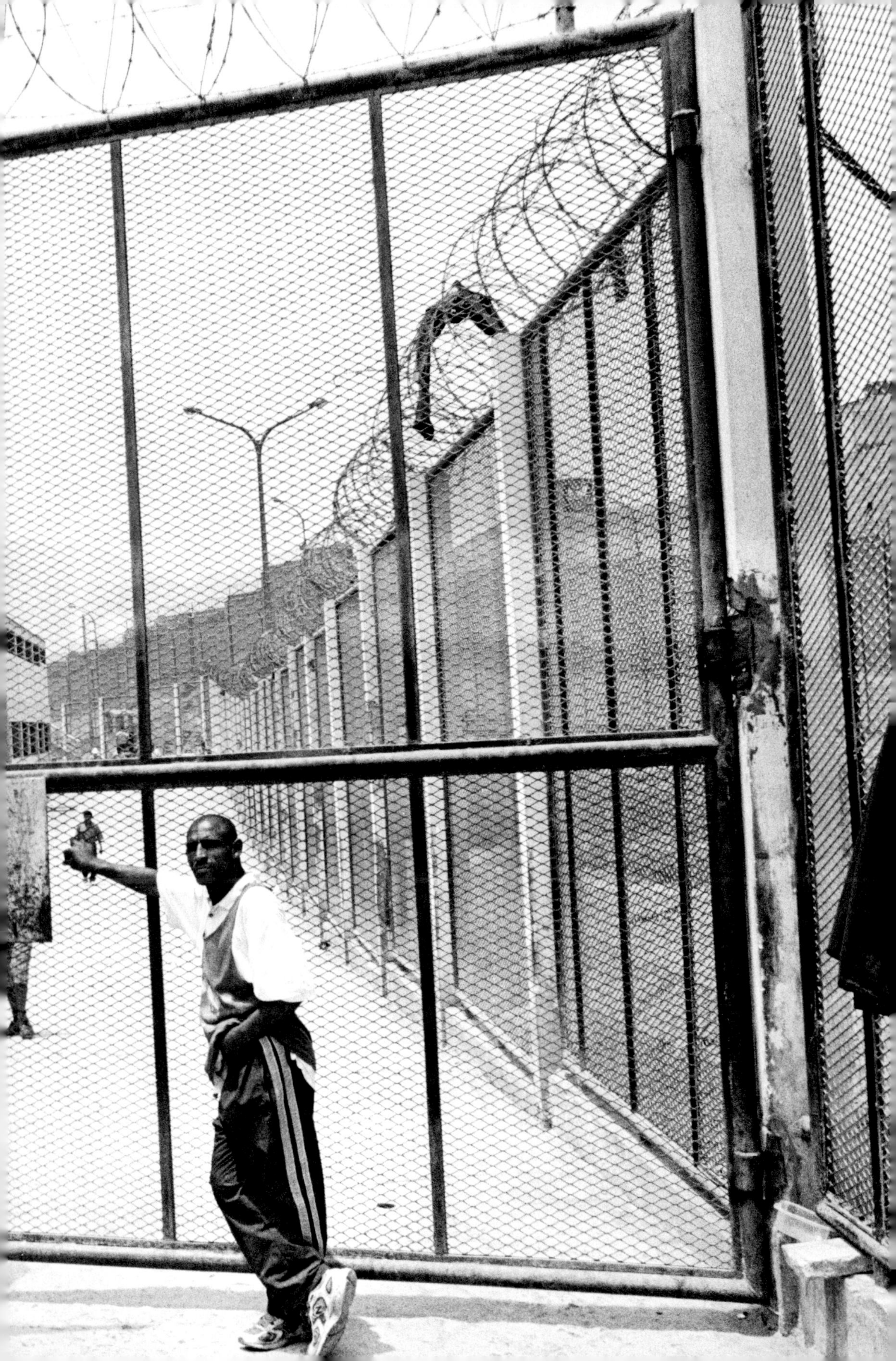

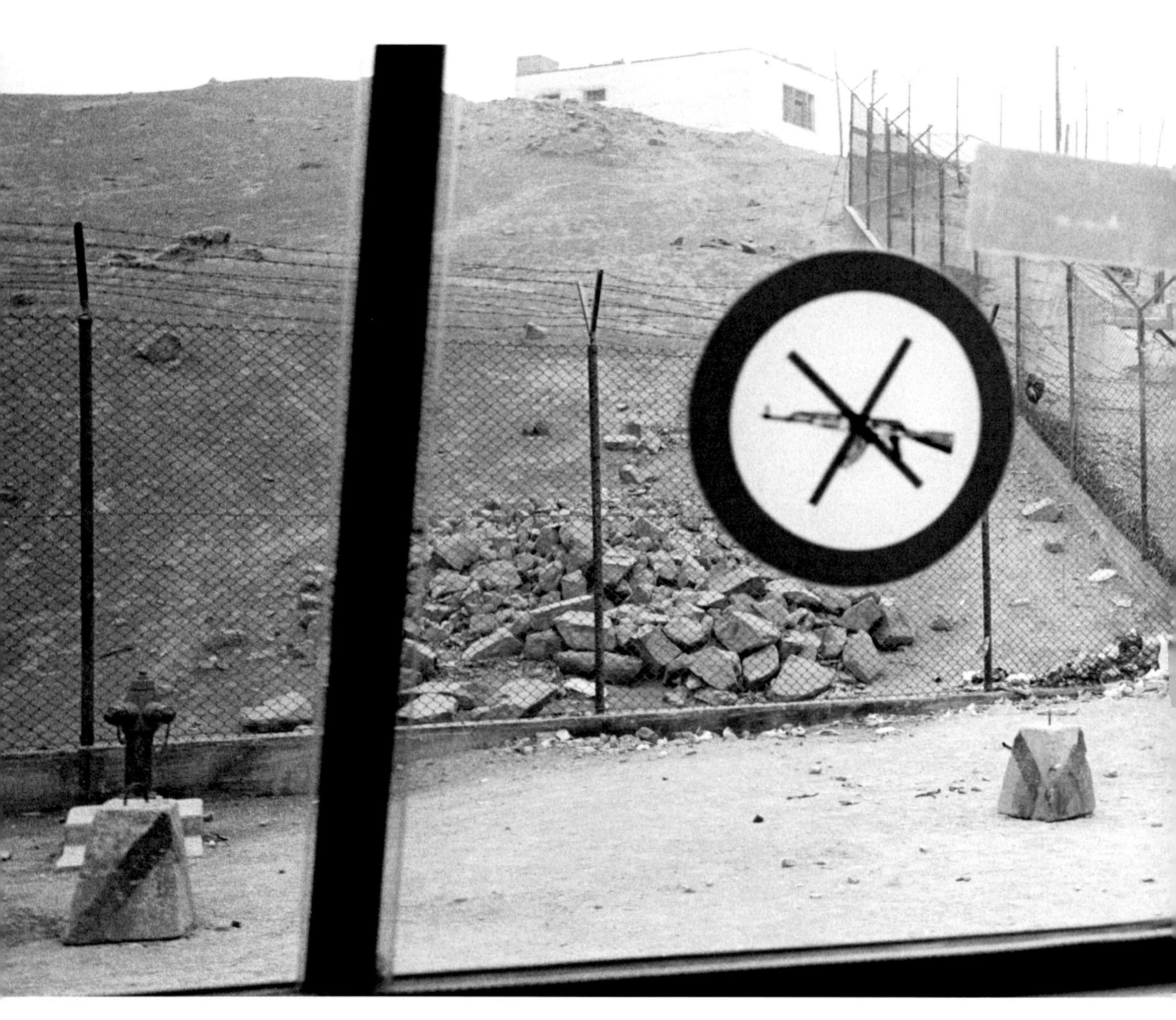

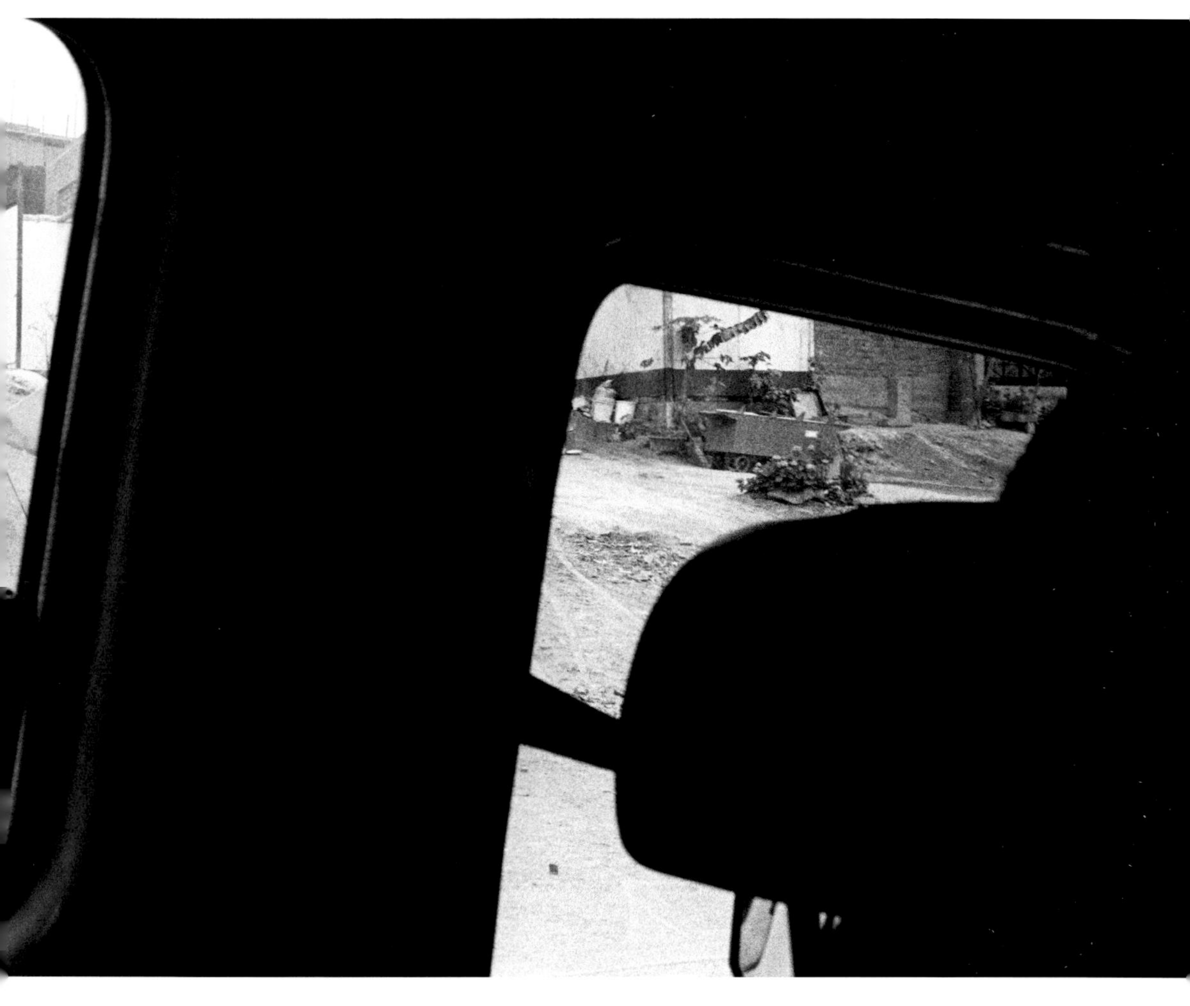

Captions

Page 2: PERU. Lima. 2006. A child who lives with her mother in a Lima slum. The child's father died of AIDS. Seven years ago, annual HIV/AIDS treatment cost $10,000. Today, a patient can be treated for less than $300 a year due to generic drugs. The total number of HIV infected persons in Peru is estimated at 93,000, with most living in the Lima and adjacent Callao area.

Page 4/5: PERU. Lima. 2006. During house visits in MSF truck. MSF Peru treats HIV/AIDS positive patients through clinics, house visits, and urban educational campaigns. Today, fewer than 5% of the 40 million world-wide AIDS victims are receiving treatment. MSF treats 23,000 patients in 27 countries.

Page 6: PERU. Lima. October 2005. Andreas is the daughter of 32-year-old AIDS patient Doris. Doris is the mother of three children and runs a small general store. Her husband died of AIDS four years ago. She attends the evangelical church "Dios Es Amor" (God Is Love) which discourages the taking of AIDS medicine as a cure.

Page 9: PERU. 2006. Lurigancho Prison. MSF doctor with AIDS patient. The risk of contracting the Human Immunodeficiency Virus (HIV) is 5 to 7 times higher in prison than on the streets. Due to the danger of an epidemic, MSF began an educational campaign and a clinic for treatment in 1998.

Page 10/11: PERU. Lima. October 2005. Windshield of MSF vehicle in Villa El Salvador, a slum neighborhood of 380,000, home to an MSF office and many of its HIV/AIDS patients. The neighborhood was once an empty field that was taken over by landless peasants who migrated to the capital in search of employment in the 1970's.

Page 15/19: PERU. Lima. 2005. Betty is 26 years old and separated from her husband, a drug addict, from whom she contracted AIDS. She and her children live with her mother.

Page 22/23: PERU. Lima. October 2005. Saturina, with medicine boxes provided by MSF. Saturina's husband died of AIDS. She lives with her three children in a slum. One of them is HIV positive.

Page 27: PERU. Lima. October 2005. Driving through Lima on house visitations to HIV/AIDS patients with "Hogar San Camilo," a Catholic relief agency run by Father Seferino. San Camilo, the organization's namesake, is the Catholic patron saint of the sick.

Page 28/29: PERU. Lima. October 2005. Red light district.

Page 30/49: PERU. Lima. 2006. Transvestite commercial sex worker. 35% of transvestites in Peru are HIV positive. 2% of "legal" and 10% of "non legal" female commercial sex workers are HIV positive.

Page 53: PERU. Lima. 2005. In an HIV patient's home during house visit.

Page 54/57: PERU. Lima. 2005. Female sex worker in brothel.

Page 61: PERU. Lima. 2005. Sex worker in a brothel during condom distribution by "Alberto Barton de Callao" sexually transmitted infection (STI) clinic.

Page 62/63: PERU. Lima. 2005. Female sex worker in brothel. 2% of "legal" and 10% of "non-legal" female commercial sex workers in Peru are HIV positive.

Page 64/65: PERU. Lima. December 1, 2006. Chorrillos (Female) Prison. Prisoners at a Catholic Mass during MSF AIDS awareness campaign at Lima's prison for women. Women may live with their babies until they are 3 years of age. There are a large number of foreigners who were caught at the airport attempting to smuggle contraband as "mules."

Page 66/67: PERU. Lima. 2006. Lurigancho Prison. Inside prison walls. Lurigancho is located at the foot of a desert hill 11 kilometres northeast of Lima's downtown.

Page 68/69: PERU. Lima. 2006. MSF team arriving at Lurigancho Prison during AIDS Awareness Week (culminating in International AIDS Day on December 1).

Page 72/77: PERU. Lima. December 1, 2006. Chorrillos (Female Prison). Women prisoners at volleyball tournament during MSF AIDS awareness campaign at Lima's prison for women. Due to the success of the campaign at Lurigancho, MSF launched a similar program at Chorrillos which houses 1040 inmates (and 12 HIV patients).

Page 78/79: PERU. Lima. 2006. Home of AIDS patient during MSF house visit in the Lomo de Coruina slum. The total number of HIV infected persons in Peru is estimated at 93,000, with most living in the Lima and adjacent Callao area.

Page 83: PERU. Lima. 2006. Lurigancho Prison. Drying laundry strung between balconies.

Page 84/85: PERU. Lima. December 1, 2006. Chorrillos (Female Prison). Women prisoners at volleyball tournament during MSF AIDS awareness campaign at Lima's prison for women.

Page 86/87: PERU. Lima. 2006. Transvestite commercial sex worker. 35% of transvestites in Peru are HIV positive. MSF Peru treats HIV/AIDS patients through clinics, house visits, and educational campaigns.

Page 88/91: PERU. Lima. 2006. Lurigancho Prison. Inside a "pavilion" (cell block).

Page 93: PERU. Lima. 2006. Lurigancho Prison. Transvestite. A particularly vulnerable population, the transvestite community in Lurigancho is nearly 50% HIV positive. Many are internal sex workers. In 1998, MSF began an HIV treatment center and an awareness campaign as it is estimated that half of prisoners have sex with other men.

Page 94/96: PERU. Lima. October 2005. Inmates at Lurigancho Prison line up for their single meal of the day during condom distribution sponsored by MSF and The Global Fund. Lurigancho is notorious for the appalling living conditions of its inmates.

Page 97: PERU. Lima. 2006. Lurigancho Prison. An inmate plays with a pet dog.

Page 98/103: PERU. Lima. 2006. Lurigancho Prison. Food preparation and men eating lunch inside pavilion. The budget allotted for food remains at about one dollar per person per day, which is inadequate for proper nutrition.Inmates must earn money to increase their ration and purchase commodities including their beds. Some prisoners eat only leftovers and have no permanent place to sleep.

Page 104/107: PERU. Lima. 2006. Lurigancho Prison. Inmates asleep. Many of those unable to pay do not have a place to sleep.

Page 108/109: PERU. Lima. 2006. Lurigancho Prison. Entrance to "pavilion" (cell block).

Page 110/111: PERU. Lima. 2006. Lurigancho Prison. Inmates during lunch.

Page 114/115: PERU. Lima. 2006. Lurigancho Prison. Inmate with pet cat.

Page 116/117: PERU. Lima. 2006. Lurigancho Prison. A transvestite barber.

Page 118/119: PERU. Lima. 2006. Lurigancho Prison. Open courtyard between "pavilions" (cell blocks).

Page 120/121: PERU. Lima. 2006. Lurigancho Prison. One of several gates separating prison sections.

Page 122/123: PERU. Lima. 2006. Lurigancho Prison. Driving in MSF vehicle outside of the prison yards.

This book has been published on the occasion of the
closure of the mission in Peru, managed for twenty
three years by Médecins Sans Frontières

The Cardboard House is the name of a novel written in 1928 by the Peruvian novelist
Rafael de la Fuente Benavides under the pseudonym Martín Adán

Published in Great Britain in 2008
By Trolley Ltd
www.trolleybooks.com

Photography © Larry Towell/ Magnum Photos
Text © MSF
Design: &&& Ltd
Text Editing: Hannah Watson, Bryony Harris

ISBN 978-1-904563-71-6

Printed in Italy 2008 by Grafiche Antiga